TOM'S LAW: FIT HAPPENS

SPEND TIME ON HEALTH, SAVE MONEY ON ILLNESS

THOMAS LAW OAM, DIP. FITNESS

Contact the author:
tomslaw@hotmail.com

The information contained in this book may help you greatly in your attempts to become fitter and healthier and enjoy a better quality of life. The book is not a medical authority. You should make sure that you consult your physician or family doctor before undergoing any physical fitness program.

ABOUT THE AUTHOR

Tom Law came to Australia as a three-year-old, from Scotland. Settling in Geraldton, Western Australia, after finishing school he completed an apprenticeship as an electrician before marrying his wife, Margaret, and joining the Australian Army.

After 21 years of service in the Royal Australian Corps of Signals, and having been awarded an Order of Australia Medal for his services to training, Thomas went back to civilian life, working in his own business, then council and eventually managing a gym.

For the last 20 years, Tom has continued his education in the health and wellness field, and works today in his own fitness business, Tom's Law.

tomslaw@hotmail.com

People and Places (2014)

Tom's Law: How to Succeed as a Personal Trainer (2017)

Dedicated to my wife and family for their patience and encouragement

The best six doctors anywhere,
And no one can deny it,
Are sunshine, water, rest, and air,
Exercise and diet.
These six will gladly you attend,
if only you are willing.
Your mind they'll ease,
your will they'll mend,
and charge you not a shilling.

NURSERY RHYME, IN WAYNE FIELDS,
WHAT THE RIVER KNOWS

CONTENTS

GROWING OLDER, STAYING YOUNG

BY DONNA DAVIS

*Well, I'm approaching three score and ten and I've
    been told that's all we get,
But the angels haven't found me, because I'm not
    finished yet.
At 61, I was old! My body creaked and groaned,
If I had to walk to the local shop (about 100m), I
    puffed and complained and moaned.*

*So I started exercise, I decided to get fit,
I had used up all the excuses, so I did a little bit.
I started aqua aerobics, even though I couldn't
    swim,
I even saw a trainer and started at the gym.*

*Then one rainy morning when I was down at
    Sutton's Beach,
I saw the strangest sight and I had a goal that I
    must reach.*

*I saw Tom Law and his boot camp, playing soccer
    in the rain,
And I thought, "This is what I want to do," so,
    ignoring all the pain,*

*I started running through the water and lifting
    weights above my head,
And crawling through the sand, and* running!
    *Something I really dread.
I didn't need a gym and fancy machines to keep
    me fit,
I just needed the park at the beach to lunge and
    squat and skip.*

*My friend is over 80 and she does push-ups by the
    score,
We're both very competitive and there's always a
    rush for the door
When we are going off to boxing or PT or boot
    camp on the beach.
For staying young and healthy is the goal for us to
    reach.*

*So if you're coming past Tom's Law, at Sutton's by
    the sea,
You'll see that age is just a state of mind, for my
    friend Lena and me.*

I started school at four years of age, and left at 15 to start an apprenticeship as an electrician. I can never remember being taken to or picked up from school apart from getting a bus ride one day from a mate's house 40km away. My sister and I walked to school together, or at least that's what our parents thought. We also walked every Saturday to the matinee at the local picture theatre and, of course, we walked home.

Even when we started work, we were seldom taken by car. I had a trusty bike that I used to get to and from work. The only real time I can remember being taken anywhere by vehicle was to soccer training and matches when Mum or Dad were available and it was convenient for them. We had a car, of course, but never a new one, and the cars we had were very unreliable and were mainly for Mum and Dad to get to work and do the shopping. It was expected that we get where we needed to by ourselves, walking, cycling or being picked up by friends. To be honest, I don't remember many cars being around in my childhood. Some of the kids I went to school with had no family car, and their parents would ride old bicycles to work. This was part of the poverty of the era, relative to today.

Everyone played some form of sport at school. It was expected that you participate. We had some reluctant kids, of course, and others who were very good, but we all attended. On sports days, every student had to enter an event. Younger kids played many games with things like beanbags[1] and hula hoops, but we graduated to athletic disciplines in later years. I played soccer and did boxing, and my sister did gymnastics. Again, we were expected to walk there and back.

I tell these stories to illustrate how the children of my generation were much more active than the children now. These are the baby boomers: people born between 1946 and 1965, give or take a year or two. The generation before that is sometimes called the Silent Generation and was probably more active again, as they had even less access to vehicles and labour-saving devices at work and in the home.

Since the baby boomers, we have had Generation X, Generation Y, Generation Z and now Generation Alpha, born from 2010 onwards, who are starting their education early and finishing later. Each generation lives in a slightly more advanced society where, I believe, labour-saving devices are encouraging us to be less active but more productive.

My father led a daily routine that was pretty much followed by most of the dads in our neighbourhood. They may have had better jobs or careers and employment, but it was my experience that most lived the same way. Dad had many jobs, ranging from labouring to office work and sales, but I can never recall him working on Saturday afternoons or Sundays.

A lot of people worked from Monday to Friday, with some working up to midday on Saturday when most businesses closed, only to reopen on Monday morning. Most people I knew worked a 40-hour week, or 44 if they worked on Saturday morning. Some convenience shops and hotels opened longer, of course, but my hometown's main street was like a ghost town on Saturday afternoons, when a lot of sport was played. Sunday was still seen as a day of rest, though the religious significance has declined over the years.

Compare my life as a child to those of the children of today, and I am sure you will agree with me that it was easier when I was a child to remain fit and healthy. Certainly, we were a lot more active, even if only by necessity. In my early days in Geraldton, Western Australia, I never dreamt I would currently be working on my third book and still be active in the industry I love.

Health and wellness to you.

Tom Law

ACKNOWLEDGMENTS

With thanks to:

Donna Davis
Daniel Law
Margaret Law
Lyn Blake
Sheila Magnier
Lesley Cooksey (Snodge)
Alison White
David Peters
Kenna Louise French
Scarborough Exercise Team
Horace Clark
Sandra and John
Marjorie Smith
Michael Flannery
Leeanne Blanckensee
Adiel Ben-Karmona
Marlene McDermid

Cathy Butter
Carmel Flett
Cheryl Springer
Heather Gibson
Ben Hourigan
Anne Macindoe

Special thanks to:

Mitch Peterman BHlthSc (Nutr. & Diet) (Hons),
BAppSc (HMS) (Hons), APD, AEP, ESSAM

WHY DID I WRITE THIS BOOK?

Being healthy comes at a small cost of your time, but being sick can be very expensive.

You may be wondering why a person whose livelihood depends on the health and wellness industry, particularly as a group and personal trainer, would write a book about how to get exercise for free. It's a reasonable question. Having been in the industry a long time, I see a cross section of the community, and know that many see health and wellness as something that can be quite expensive. I can almost hear my late mum saying, "It may be well and good to spend time and money on sport and exercise, but that doesn't put food on the table." That's true, but I know writing this book won't make people leave gyms and personal trainers in droves. In fact, it's likely to do the reverse. The book may encourage people to do more about getting regular exercise, and to be a little more thoughtful about how they eat. I genuinely would like to see more people exercising regularly. The benefits are well and truly worth it.

A long time ago, someone told me to always remember to put back into the community. My family and I have been lucky. Of course, we worked hard, like most people who end up reasonably comfortable in life, but many work hard and still never seem to get the lucky breaks. I did get some lucky breaks, and so have other members of my family, and for that I am very grateful. I look around at people I admire in the local community who give their time and, in some cases, significant sums of money to help people and causes that need it. My family and I also like to contribute, and we do, in ways that we think are appropriate and within our means.

One way I've been able to contribute is through my work. My business, Tom's Law, has always provided exercise for those who cannot afford it. We might let them exercise free with our group, and we've conducted free exercise programs in the community. I believe my responsibility as a health provider is to help where I can. Of course, I run a business and money is paramount, but helping people to be fit and healthy is something princes and paupers alike should have access to. This book, I am hopeful, will contribute to the community by educating those who need it to the ways in which exercise can be undertaken for very little cost and, in many cases, completely free.

In my experience, there are three types of people who exercise: the gym user, the outdoor exerciser or boot camp attendee, and the free exerciser. Now, there are permutations, variations and combinations, and there may be more categories, but I think most fit into those three.

I work every day in the health and wellness field, not as a medical practitioner, physiotherapist, nurse or dietician, but as a personal trainer. I am both inspired and disappointed daily by the cross section of people I come across in an attempt to help them to become healthier.

Those people who work with me or any other personal trainer or health professional, who are trying to become healthier, stronger, fitter, faster and so on, impress and encourage me, and remind me every day of the reason I love this job. But I also see people who are obviously not doing all they can to help themselves have a more productive and generally healthier lifestyle. This disappoints me. I find it hard to understand how, given choices in life, people still choose to take a road that in many instances leads to constant medical care, hospitalisation and even worse. Of course, as the saying goes, "We don't survive this life," but given the chance, wouldn't most people want to live as healthily as they could for as long as possible? I really believe that, with a little prodding and a lot of encouragement, many people can be convinced to change their habits and pursue a healthier way of life.

One of the reasons I wrote this book is to help those people who want to help themselves. I hope you enjoy it and, more importantly, I hope it helps you become healthier so you can enjoy all the benefits that flow from that.

Several years ago, the expression "ambulance at the bottom of the cliff" caught my attention. A politician used it to describe the way we treat the fallout of people hooked on illegal drugs, by providing support and medical measures rather than preventive measures. I don't want to put words in his mouth; he did mention we allocate money for prevention but a lot is used in support and rehabilitation. The thing that impressed me was how evocative that comment was. In Australia, we do a lot to help people help themselves regarding health and wellness, especially if they've fallen off a cliff, but I'm not convinced we're doing enough to keep them from going over the edge.

We spend plenty of money on community facilities like running tracks, parks, and exercise stations and, if you're lucky to have a local council like I do in my area, even free exercise programs. How good is that? In Australia, we are lucky that governments at all levels are interested in providing free facilities and exercise opportunities for us. And from my travels, I must admit that China seems to be doing the same, if not more, to help the locals keep fit, with free park facilities on a very large scale.

So why do I believe it is not enough?

Well, let's take China for example. Although I am not a local or an expert on China, I've holidayed there, and I can see the irony that the same government that provides great exercise facilities for its citizens has let the air become so thick with pollution that some days you can't see from one side of the street to the other. (I do acknowledge that China now seems to be doing a lot of work to combat pollution.) And in Australia, our hospitals are full of people with diabetes and heart disease, which the experts tell us are preventable. A lot of people from overseas must think it strange that a modern country like Australia, with great weather, fantastic beaches and an abundance of fresh food and water, has an alarming obesity rate. I know *I* think it is strange.

In 2014/15, more than one in four adult Australians were obese. This represents almost five million Australians aged 18 and over (BMI of 30.0kg/m² or more). More than two million

Australian men were obese, or approximately 28% of all males aged 18 and over. Close to 2.5 million Australian women were obese, or approximately 27% of all females aged 18 and over.[1]

The way we live is full of contradictions, and this is one area where I believe our government can do more. We sell cigarettes, then treat the conditions they cause. We let companies peddle addictive drinks full of flavouring and sugar, then treat the fallout of obesity-related diseases and diabetes. The amount of advertising money spent on alcohol promotion must be obscene, while alcohol-related health issues directly and indirectly take a toll on our health system. But all the above is typical of a free country. We may be able to sell unhealthy products, but it's not compulsory to consume them. So *the consequences really come down to the choices we make.*

The medical profession and scientific research have made amazing discoveries, and these advances are allowing us to live longer, but will we live better if we don't address some of the big health issues?

We can do something. First, we can take some personal responsibility and actively participate in the health revolution. We can put pressure on those who supply unhealthy products by refusing to buy them. Years ago, the Australian government decided to wage war on cigarette consumption. They did this over many years, and it worked. Cigarette smoking in Australia, according to the Bureau of Statistics, dropped from 28.2% in 2001 to 16.3% in 2014. Although cigarettes are still sold, a massive anti-smoking education program has had some traction.

We can have a similar impact if we refuse to buy unhealthy products. Manufacturers get the message and adapt or disappear. We have seen the healthy trend continue in Australia, with many large fast food companies changing their product line-up to include healthy, fresh options, so we can see the power of the people does work, though sometimes slowly. One of the ways I think more can be done is in a concerted public awareness program, like the very successful campaign against cigarette smoking a number of years ago in Australia. Another controversial advertising campaign that had a fantastic public response was the electronic media's AIDS advertisements. Both the Life Be In It and AIDS awareness campaigns had a fantastic response from the public, and perhaps a concerted effort towards healthier eating and more regular exercise could be just as effective.

Second, keeping in mind that the main focus of this book is your health, you will not only do yourself a big favour by looking after it, but will also have a positive influence on those around you. Your family, workmates and friends will respond to your positive approach to health and fitness. We often underestimate the power of a positive role model or mentor. You may not always be aware of the effect you have on some people, but good habits can be contagious. You may not have to say anything; leading by example may be good enough.

Exercise should not have to cost you anything more than the price of appropriate clothes to wear and a good set of exercise running or cross training shoes. I have always believed that, and I live my life this way, though my business is based on people paying to be provided with exercise. I know many people need motivation and encouragement, and that may be provided by a personal trainer like myself, or in a gym. But if you have the right attitude and motivation, you can do it all yourself. One of the main aims of this book is to encourage you to lead a generally healthier life.

I have travelled around Australia, and have been impressed by the free facilities cities and towns provide for locals and visitors to help keep them fit and healthy for free. I have also used similar equipment overseas, and would say that the equipment provided abroad and at home seldom looks overused. In many cases, the opposite is true.

In case suitable fixed exercise stations or open spaces and parks are not available where you live, I will show you how to adapt and improvise to help improve your overall health. I will encourage you to get out and use whatever facilities you have at your disposal. You will also be able to use this book as a valuable resource and training guide. There is no need for you to buy expensive equipment or spend lots of money on gym memberships unless you want to. All you will ever need is in this book. The basics of health and wellness are well and truly tried and tested. Of course, we will see new trends regularly and modern research will fine-tune all aspects of health and fitness. This can only be a good thing.

My wife always tells me we have choices in life. We can choose to be as healthy as we can, given our circumstances, or we can ignore our health. It is entirely feasible that a poor person with very little money and personal possessions can, by choice, be healthier, fitter and happier than a millionaire. We see that throughout the world. The choice, in many instances, is ours to make. I am convinced you will be happier and healthier, and live much better in many ways, if you strive to strike a balance in your life that includes sensible eating and regular exercise.

Keep this book handy. There are guidelines and references in here that cover essential basics such as recommended waist measurements and BMI (body mass index) values, and recommended physical activity. I have highlighted this information for you in bold print for ease of use. You will find this book contains all the basic information you will ever need to keep yourself fit, healthy and in good physical shape.

If you follow these guidelines, you will be able to become fit and maintain your fitness, which will help your overall health and wellness. You may not necessarily live longer, but you have a terrific chance of living a lot better. It really is very simple. Your small investment in this book may change your life and save you plenty of money. Enjoy the journey.

CHAPTER ONE
SOME SCIENCE FIRST

When I read a book, I want to get to the exciting part quickly. More than a few times, I've flicked a page or skipped a paragraph or even a chapter to get to the meaty part. I mention that because you're about to read some statistics provided by the Australian Government Department of Health, which may seem dry to most of us but are an important part of the overall picture about health and wellness. The information highway these days is enormously wide, and you can get any amount of literature about health. It's easy to get confused. I prefer to use what I can get from organisations like government departments whose research is proven, consistent and accurate.

PHYSICAL ACTIVITY GUIDELINES (FROM THE AUSTRALIAN GOVERNMENT DEPARTMENT OF HEALTH)

- Doing any physical activity is better than doing none. If you currently do no physical activity, start by doing

some, and gradually build up to the recommended
amount.
- Be active on most, preferably all days every week.
- Accumulate 150 to 300 minutes (2½ to 5 hours) of
  moderate intensity physical activity or 75 to
  150 minutes (1¼ to 2½ hours) of vigorous intensity
  physical activity, or an equivalent combination of
  both moderate and vigorous activities, each week.
- Do muscle strengthening activities on at least two
  days each week.[1]

These guidelines are for people in Australia aged 18 to 64. I
find this site particularly good as a guide because it recommends activity for most age groups. It is a handy, well-
researched and concise reference—but I have also
summarised much of the relevant information here for your
convenience.

The Mayo Clinic believes that exercise helps in the following
areas:

- controlling weight
- combating health conditions and diseases
- improving mood
- boosting energy
- promoting better sleep
- putting the spark back into your sex life
- fostering fun and social engagement[2]

In his book *The Aerobics Program for Total Well-Being*, Dr
Kenneth Cooper, known as the father of aerobics, wrote:

"Just to give you a taste of what can happen in your life, here are some of the benefits of total well-being that data from our research has shown us can be yours for the asking:

- More personal energy;
- More enjoyable and active leisure time;
- Greater ability to handle domestic and job-related stress;
- Less depression, less hypochondria and less "free-floating" anxiety;
- Fewer physical complaints;
- More efficient digestion and fewer problems with constipation;
- A better self-image and more self-confidence;
- A more attractive, streamlined body, including more effective personal weight control;
- Bones of greater strength;
- Slowing of the aging process;
- Easier pregnancy and childbirth;
- More restful sleep;
- Better concentration at work, and greater perseverance in all daily tasks;
- Fewer aches and pains, including back pain."[3]

Now, I could go on and, in fact, you will find additional health benefits listed in further chapters to reinforce the amazing benefits of regular exercise and good nutrition. I am sure you get the point. In all my time in this business, I don't recall anyone saying exercise is bad for you. I would be exceptionally surprised to hear that, and think that as even more labour-saving devices are invented and introduced into society, much more importance will be placed on exercise and movement.

Females born from 2015 to 2017 can expect to live around four years longer than males—84.6 years compared with 80.5 years.[4]

There is no doubting that science, improvements and discoveries in the field of medicine, and better education are benefiting many of us. How we live those additional years to some extent may be directly up to us and the way we choose to live our lives.

Enough facts about our health and wellness. Let's look at how we get our exercise now, in the modern world. To do this, it is only fair that we look back and see how things have changed and how much harder it is for many of us to get our recommended exercise requirements in every week. It's a personal thing, of course, but most people decide to start living healthier at some stage of their lives. Generally, this realisation comes after the exuberance of youth but before retirement.

Many of us accept the notion that generally we don't do enough to keep ourselves healthy with regular exercise. The world is different from what it used to be. In the very short time from my childhood to today, the changes, improvements and advancements have been amazing. My father, and his father before him, may have said the same. Few of us now need to do hard physical labour, and though there are certainly many of these types of jobs still around, fantastic advances in technology have reduced the physical strain.

One example that comes readily to mind is the long-gone dustman, who would normally hang off the back of a truck while it crawled up the street in the early hours of the morning. At each house, the man would jump off the truck, run into your yard to grab your metal bin, run back out to the truck and empty the contents. He would then return your empty bin to the place he found it, and repeat this process for every house in the street. Compare that to the modern era: the bin is now plastic, considerably larger and on wheels, and you simply place it on the kerb where a truck with a mechanical arm performs the same operation a man performed many years ago. The energetic, slim and fit dustman of my childhood has been replaced by a sedentary truck driver who seldom gets out of his cab. It was not uncommon for a boxer, footballer or sportsman of some sort to seek employment in a job like this to enhance their training in days gone by. Unfortunately for them, that type of physical effort is not required anymore.

The workmen of yesteryear never seemed too far away from a tool like a shovel or sledgehammer for doing all sorts of things, from digging holes in the street to fixing leaking water pipes or demolishing buildings. These people have often been replaced by machines, and often, the person driving those machines have a slightly thicker waistline. Not everyone is like this, but you get the picture.

Now let's look at office workers, who in years past may have ridden a bike, walked or used public transport to get to work, but now mainly drive to work. I often recall my friends' fathers riding their pushbikes to work. My grandmother, each weekday, would walk two miles to work as a cleaner at a school, and then walk two miles back. I remember this well, as from time to time I served as her little assistant, particularly during school holidays.

According to the Australian Bureau of Statistics, as of 2008:

Although there has been a slight increase in the use of public transport over the past 10 years, in March 2006, three-quarters (75%) of adults living in capital cities travelled to their usual place of work or study using private motor vehicles as their main form of transport. In addition, 19% of adults used public transport, and a further 5% either walked or cycled as their main form of transport to work or study.[5]

Even the office environment has changed, becoming more automated and high-tech. Opportunities for exercise have reduced significantly. More and more employees in high-rise buildings are being excluded from using the stairs, which are now seen as for emergency use only and fitted with alarms. The main reason for this is to increase security from theft, reducing the risk that people will use the fire escape stairs to get away. Most buildings will let you leave the building at the ground level without any problem, but you cannot enter another floor from a fire escape, or, obviously, enter the building using the fire escape stairs at ground level. The opportunities to get exercise at work are also being reduced due to technological advances. I cannot see any boss being happy for employees to walk down 20 flights of stairs on a daily basis just to stretch their legs, outside of their programmed breaks.

At home, it has been a long time since we had to get up and walk a few paces to turn the TV on and off, or even to change channels. Many people reading this book may not even give much thought to how TVs were not always operated remotely. It's easy to forget about these things. Food can now be delivered to your door with after just a few minutes spent on a phone call or mobile app. Laundry requires virtually no effort beyond loading the machine. House cleaning used to be a solid manual workout, involving scrubbing floors and plenty of elbow grease. Modernisation has changed that somewhat. The vacuum cleaner, dishwasher, carpeted floors, modern bathroom materials and self-cleaning ovens are just a few present-day conveniences that make the job of cleaning a house less strenuous.

Recently, I was pumping up my car tyre. The rear left-hand tyre has a very slow leak. Because of the balls we use at exercise, I carry a car pump in my work van, and during a break between personal training sessions, I decided to pump up the tyre manually. Another gentleman at a car park nearby drove up to me and kindly offered me his pneumatic electric pump. I declined graciously and told him I really preferred to get a little workout manually by pumping up the tyre. Most people would consider that strange. I don't.

A week or so ago, I was walking the 1.2km from my unit to a restaurant in the town where I live. During the walk, some of my clients came past in a car. They were going to the same restaurant, so they stopped to offer me a lift. I thanked them but declined, and told them I was making sure I got my daily allocation of steps. I am sure they could not believe I wouldn't take the lift, and I'd imagine not many people would decline the offer. I simply wanted to enjoy my walk and get in some exercise. Is it so hard to believe that we could enjoy walking?

I could go on, but the message is clear: we now need to plan and program our exercise because more and more, we are doing less and less. Don't get me wrong, plenty of readers will be so very grateful for the advances in technology and the labour-saving devices we now have, and so am I, but the fact remains that we are doing less physical activity in our normal everyday routine.

Later in this book (chapter 6), I talk about "incidental exercise", which is the exercise you get as a part of your day without specifically aiming to exercise. Incidental exercise, or the rate at which we get it, has decreased in direct proportion to the number of modern-day inventions that profess to make our day easier and give us more time to do other things. Many of our modern-day appliances and machinery have saved us labour, but have also taken away a lot of our daily opportunities for movement.

Chapter 10 includes some more technical information on BMI, waist measurements and heart rate that you may also find useful as you embark on your journey to better health and wellness.

CHAPTER TWO
THE BENEFITS OF KEEPING HEALTHY

How long is a piece of string? It's a common response to questions that can't be answered easily.

What are the benefits of keeping healthy? How long is a piece of string? I could write a whole book on the topic, and it seems every day another luminary, scholar or scientist comes up with even more reasons why it is so important to keep healthy. Health may come as a physical, mental or spiritual thing but, in this book, we are only concentrating on improving physical health through exercise and good nutrition. The benefits of keeping physically healthy are numerous, and I will list and discuss many of them in this chapter, though they are likely countless.

Humans started out as very efficient machines, hunting and gathering food and drink to stay alive. Our bodies were lean, and our major focus between meals was survival, or where the next meal would come from. Fast-forward to today, and most of us work in sedentary jobs. The hunger is literally not there, and we don't have to be as efficient a machine as our Stone Age counterparts did. We've become soft. Not all of us, that's true, but not all of us are as healthy and as fit as we could be.

In the previous chapter, I listed some of the benefits of exercise that Dr Kenneth Cooper and the Mayo Clinic have high-lighted. Here I expand a bit with some real examples of people who have benefited from adjusting their exercise and health regime, or who have started a healthier living routine.

The best strategy I have come across for explaining the benefits of being healthy is simple but effective: compare your body to a machine like a motor vehicle. If you keep your car in good order, get it serviced on time and keep it well maintained, the chances are it will serve you well. If you make sure you put in the correct lubricants and top-quality fuel, it will also perform at its maximum capacity. Your body is very similar. Keep your body well maintained, the circulation moving—with plenty of water and good food and an absolute minimum of rubbish—and your body will work well. Your motor vehicle and body both need maintenance and great additives, on a regular basis.

One of the tools for measuring how healthy we are is how you feel. Most people I know who want to be healthier, if not fitter, tell me they are not happy with their body and don't feel good. They may be carrying a bit more weight, feel out of breath when playing with the kids, want to be stronger or even need to lose weight before they can have children.

How are you with doing simple daily physical activities like bending over to do up your shoelaces? Is it becoming increas-ingly harder? What about getting dressed in the morning? Can you put on your underwear or socks without sitting down on the bed? Do you still have the dexterity and balance to do some of these simple daily tasks? When did you last see your toes when you looked down in the shower? Is your tummy in the way? Can you still touch your toes?

If you can still do all these things, good for you. If not, I am sure I will be able to help you. Read on.

If you speak to your doctor, family, friends or personal trainer, everyone has different reasons why you should keep healthy and fit. All of them are probably correct, but to me, the number one reason is this: we keep fit and healthy to stay physically and mentally active for as long as possible, and for a good quality of life. Naturally, with that comes good strength and aerobic capacity, balance and mental alertness, and many other desirable abilities. My reason for wanting to maintain good health and fitness is so I can interact with my grandchildren for as long as possible. I am sure you have your own reasons, and good for you. Keeping healthy and active gives you the best chance of being able to do what you want to for longer. Of that, there is no doubt.

As I was writing this chapter, I wondered whether I should list all those things that being healthy helps with. Instead, I will give a few examples of people I know through my business and exercise program who have improved their health and life-style. You may find you can relate to their stories.

Of course, the list of benefits of keeping healthy could fill a chapter or even a whole book. Between the last chapter and this one, I cover a fair bit of ground on the benefits of keeping healthy. The amazing thing with good health is there are no bad or side effects. It is all positive. We don't get out of this life alive, but how good would it be to remain free from illness and active for as long as possible? The stories that follow show you how it's possible to get much closer to that goal.

YOUR ATTITUDE CAN CHANGE

Let's take Julie as the first case. Julie came to me several years ago when I was managing a gym. She was around 50 at the time, a single woman with no major health issues and no stressful family situations. She had a well-paying and stable job, and attended a gym three to four times per week. Her fitness and weight had plateaued, but she still wanted to lose a few more pounds and become a bit fitter.

After I talked to Julie and did a full health assessment, we worked out that the only thing Julie was doing to excess was drinking wine. Living alone, Julie would often open and finish a bottle of wine each night, and although this was her only vice, it was also one she could change.

I changed Julie's program to suit this goal and ensured her progress was monitored. I also suggested she attend at least one PT (personal training) session a week. She improved to the extent that her home drinking habits changed, and her attitude to exercise changed with a new program too. It was therefore no surprise that she met and maintained her goals.

I moved on from that gym a year or so later, and have since lost touch with Julie, but her story has been repeated many times in my experience, and there is no reason why you cannot similarly find comfort and contentment in achieving your health goals if you apply yourself. Sometimes the changes are relatively subtle or minor, but they can have an enormously positive effect on your health and well-being.

And as with Julie, there is still no reason why you cannot have the occasional glass of wine—just not a whole bottle.

EXERCISE CAN HELP DIABETICS

George had Type 2 diabetes, technically called diabetes mellitus. In this type, the body has difficulty producing enough insulin, which normally helps the body direct glucose to the muscles and liver, and assists with the storage of nutrients. When the body does not produce insulin in sufficient quantities, in most cases medication is needed to help the body perform the above functions.

This is only general information, and you should seek medical advice if you are or suspect you may be a diabetic.

More than 50% of Type 2 diabetics can significantly reduce the amount of medication they need and in many instances, if they manage their condition properly, can eliminate it entirely. Management here means a controlled diet and an appropriate, well-thought-out exercise program.

Now, back to George. George wanted to become fitter and healthier, and at no stage did we discuss reducing his medication intake. In fact, coming off medication was not one of his goals. But it did happen, though not by design. I built George a program I thought would suit him and asked him to attend the gym three times a week. I also gave him additional exercises to complete at home. He did all this religiously.

Within three months of starting his exercise program, George was not only showing good signs via his VO_2 max tests,[1] but his sugar levels were also falling. I cannot be 100% sure of the time frame, but believe it was around six months from the start of his exercise program that George was told he no longer required medication for Type 2 diabetes. What a great result!

George is not the first diabetic I know who has adjusted their lifestyle to include diet and exercise and eventually come off medication. I must stress, though, that this is an individual thing, and the need for medication must be assessed by a medical professional. I am also aware that not all Type 2 diabetics will succeed in reducing or eliminating medication. While diet and a measured exercise program will no doubt assist, elimination of medication is not guaranteed in all cases. My wife is also a Type 2 diabetic, and she has been told that although she exercises and has a healthy diet, she may not come off medication. She comes from a long line of diabetics, and her chances of becoming a diabetic were greatly increased simply by genetics.

EXERCISE CAN MAKE YOU LOOK GOOD

Jennifer is a young, well-educated woman. She came to me to help her to fit into her wedding dress. Jennifer was slight anyway, but I devised a plan to help her. She eventually lost 10kg and fit into her wedding dress perfectly, well before her wedding date. I know of many women who would be so happy to have the physique and apparent fitness levels that Jennifer started with before her weight loss, but this simply proves that health and well-being are relative to the individual.

It is about what you want, not what someone else sees or wants for you. You need to feel good about your body and body image to be completely happy. I should add that Jennifer worked very hard and was single-minded about exercising and achieving her goal. Jennifer is now happily married, and still exercises at least four times per week to maintain her physique and health and fitness.

EXERCISE CAN HELP YOU MAINTAIN MOBILITY

As I have already mentioned, the list of benefits that come from being fit could almost fill a separate book. My own experience of maintaining a good level of health and fitness means I can still operate as a very active fitness instructor in my sixties. I am not as capable as I was when younger, obviously, but I am a lot wiser and know many things now that I didn't know then. I can pace myself better, I seldom get sick and, if I do, I tend to shake it off quickly. I work every day, not a full day, but nonetheless I do work every day. I still get up every morning at 3.45am, ready to go. I do take the opportunity to get a little nap in the middle of the day if I can, as I start early and work late most days. I feel terrific and put it all down to maintaining a positive outlook on life and living a moderate and healthy lifestyle with plenty of exercise. You can do the same; perhaps you already are.

HEALTHY PEOPLE TAKE FEWER SICK DAYS

In my exercise groups, there are several people who operate large family businesses, as well as middle and upper-level managers of large corporations. All these people tell me that the fitter, healthier people in their companies have less absenteeism due to illness.

This makes sense to me, and although I have seen similar things in my own workplace, I cannot find statistics to confirm this. What I do know is that those owners, CEOs and supervisors who attend my exercise classes believe a fitter employee is not only happier, but also tends to take fewer sick days than an employee who is not as fit and therefore, it is assumed, does not exercise regularly.

I have had owners from two companies pay in advance for their own employees to attend exercise classes I ran simply to improve their fitness and well-being. I am sure the bosses were also hopeful that a healthier employee would become a better attendee at work and productivity would be increased.

YOUR SEX LIFE MAY IMPROVE

One of my clients, who attends group training, told me he thought his sex life had improved dramatically with his regular attendance at exercise. His weight had reduced, he had more get up and go, and he had a lot more endurance. It makes sense—why wouldn't it? Once again, this is an observation that may be hard to prove generally, but when you think about it, one would think having more energy would be beneficial in many everyday life situations, including relationships.

In his case, and I am sure in many more, keeping healthy was great for my client's relationship.

YOUR BODY WORKS BETTER AND MORE EFFICIENTLY

We were all shocked a few years ago to learn that one of our regular attendees, around 60 years of age, had a stroke at work. Luckily, he was attended to immediately, received fantastic medical support and was released from hospital in a matter of three days.

We wondered how this could happen to such a fit man, but were told that the stroke was associated with a recent medical procedure. Having suffered it, he was in and out of hospital so quickly simply because he was so fit and resilient. His body was efficient and worked so well it basically healed him, along with the latest science and technology. "Heal yourself" is a phrase I like. I honestly believe a positive outlook in life, combined with good eating habits and a healthy body, can go a long way to helping to heal you when you take ill.

YOU RECOVER QUICKER WHEN YOU ARE HEALTHIER

I want to highlight the benefits of exercise in two clients' recovery from injury and surgery.

One of my clients tore his Achilles tendon while playing football. After treatment, he could only walk using crutches, and the process for recovery included a long rehabilitation period complete with a moon boot. Complete recovery depends on a number of things, but a positive outlook and good fitness levels are crucial for a speedier mend. My client not only recovered quickly, but both he and his doctor attributed that quicker recovery to his continuing to exercise during the rehabilitation period. Obviously, the exercise was limited and specific, and conducted in consultation with a physiotherapist, but it advanced the process.

Another client, after years of being in pain and not having the total freedom he wanted, not to mention carrying added weight around his waist, decided at 60 years of age to bite the bullet and have both knees replaced at the same time. I am not exaggerating when I tell you that two weeks after the operation, his surgeon was amazed at his progress. The surgeon, my client and I all put it down to the fact that he exercised, within his limitations, right up to the time of his operation. None of us has any doubt that his recovery process was faster simply because of that exercise.

Having been in this field for many years, I have hundreds of examples of people where exercise and better health have positively affected people's lives. I am sure the stories above, and similar ones you may know of, will reinforce my point about the massive gains to be had in maintaining a healthy lifestyle with regular exercise.

Life is movement; keep moving.

YOU HAVE AN IMPROVED MENTAL STATE

The feel-good factor is a big benefit of exercise. I see it all the time in my industry. Ladies regain their waistline or, at least become happier with it, and their general posture improves. Exercise can do that. Men start to build muscle again. Though we know that as we age it becomes harder to build muscle quickly, it is possible.

The confidence associated with being fit cannot be overstated. Those who have recently come back to exercise, or who start for the first time, report a sense of well-being and confidence. When you feel confident, you look good, and some even take a little more care of themselves. It's a great feeling, which can so easily be achieved naturally with a little effort, dedication, motivation and application. Even if you're not achieving your goals as quickly as you want to, when you start exercise, just knowing you are on the journey towards achieving the goals you have set is a great incentive and confidence-booster.

In 2016, the Queensland Brain Institute at the University of Queensland began a study with older adults involving exercise and the effects it has on the body and brain. The study encouraged people from ages 65 to 85 to become more physically active, participate in regular exercise programs, be part of a supportive community and learn more about brain health and memory. The research confirmed that exercise was able to increase production of new brain cells and improve learning and memory.

Over the years, I have had some clients with PTSD (post-traumatic stress disorder) attend our sessions. All of them have told me that exercise not only provides a distraction from their troubles, but also helps their state of mind for some time afterwards. One middle-aged lady told me she was suffering from a form of depression or PTSD. This lady had been exercising with me for over five years and I had no idea. One evening after class, she confided in me that after an aerobic boxing session, she was on a natural high for three days. The positive effect exercise had on this lady helped her deal with any issues she had on a daily basis. How good is that? In her case, there was no need for medication. Exercise was enough for her to be on top of the world, even if only for a few days.

A husband-and-wife team attended my sessions several years ago. The husband suffered from depression, and both of them told me he benefited from exercise and felt his mood was much better if he exercised a few times a week. The feel-good factor that comes from regular exercise cannot be underestimated.

A personal trainer I know is having very positive results with her exercise program designed for multiple-sclerosis patients. MS is a disease of the central nervous system, and this trainer has designed an aerobic boxing program that is having fantastic results on her clients' balance and sense of well-being. The program is not a permanent fix, of course, but her clients are getting a much-needed boost to their health and confidence.

YOU FEEL MUCH BETTER

You can feel better when you exercise and eat properly. It may seem like you feel lighter, stronger and more alert, or you find you have a lot more energy. The sense of wellness that comes from eating sensibly and exercising regularly may be different for different people. I have never had anyone tell me they did not feel good in some way as a result. I know from my own experience that if I keep up a healthy diet and exercise, I feel really good, light and full of energy. People who exercise with me report a sense of wellness and a feeling of being lighter and more energetic when they eat and drink sensibly.

Later, I will discuss a bit more about what constitutes eating well, and we have a whole chapter by Mitch Peterman, a dietitian, on food and how we need never to diet again. For now, think about how you feel when you overeat. You may feel bloated, heavy and unhealthy, and exercise is the last thing on your mind. The opposite is true when your food intake is sensible and you have a regular exercise program. It really is simple.

EXERCISE CAN RELIEVE STRESS

Exercise can relieve stress. Many people who exercise do so to become healthier and fitter, but a by-product of that can be the reduction of stress. Many have told me they use exercise as a stress reliever. Just concentrating on something else for a time can make a big difference in people's lives. But from a purely physical point of view, being fitter means your heart rate is slower. When you become stressed and anxious, this rate increases. However, a fit and conditioned heart tends to increase its rate only marginally, where the unconditioned heart may race and cause anxiety through the changes in the body. This is the fight or flight response. Regular exercise slows the heart rate by building heart muscle and the capacity to pump more blood efficiently. So being fitter can often make you calmer and less stressed when it counts. Don't just take my word for it: numerous studies confirm this. The following statement is from the American College of Sports Medicine:

> Exercise can be an effective component of a stress management program, and all types of exercise can be beneficial for stress *management*. Exercise programs, consistent with the current recommendations to improve health, can be prescribed to manage stress.[2]

The Australian Government Department of Health states:

it is important to gradually start increasing the amount of exercise you do. This is an important part of stress management. Aim for three sessions of exercise per week, choosing activities that you enjoy and varying the types of exercise so that you are able to establish and maintain a routine.[3]

YOU SET THE EXAMPLE

Before I leave this chapter, I want to mention one other positive outcome of a healthy lifestyle. You set a great example for your family and those in your immediate circle. It is no secret that mums and dads are great role models, and anything that is done in a family setting can and will influence your children. Even if you are not married or in a relationship, you may be a teacher, boss, friend or family member. Your actions are often mimicked, which is something that parents are very aware of or should be. Your habits, be they good or bad, will influence those close to you, even some who are not so close. I still vividly remember a couple of people who impressed me at school for various reasons, but mainly because I looked up to them as role models.

One of my close friends who started out with me as a client, and a very large one at that, told me he wanted to be slimmer, fitter and healthier for several reasons. One of the main ones was so he could be a great role model for his children. The way you bring up your children, and the influence you have on them has a big bearing on how they live and how they end up parenting themselves. The fact is, you are a role model, even if you may not think about it too much. You are being watched, copied and admired, even though you may not be aware of it.

Being a good role model for your children and grandchildren, and those you mentor, teach or coach, includes every facet of life. Leading a healthy, active lifestyle is just as infectious as good manners and great behaviour.

I think it only fair and accurate to mention that you can be a great role model at any age, for people of any age. I not only think I am a good role model for my grandchildren, but also believe they are good role models for me in some instances.

- Doing any physical activity is better than doing none. If you currently do no physical activity, start by doing some, and gradually build up to the recommended amount.
- Be active on most, preferably all days every week.
- Accumulate 150 to 300 minutes (2½ to 5 hours) of moderate intensity physical activity or 75 to 150 minutes (1¼ to 2½ hours) of vigorous intensity physical activity, or an equivalent combination of both moderate and vigorous activities, each week.
- Do muscle strengthening activities on at least two days each week.[1]

This was taken straight out of the physical guidelines from the Australian Government Department of Health that I mentioned in the previous chapter, and I repeat the advice because it is so important. This is all you need to do to keep fit and healthy. So how about equipment, gym memberships and so on? What do you need to achieve that level of activity?

One of the things that encouraged me to write this book was the confusion that exists among my own clients about how to exercise and what you need to do so. The amount of information now available to us all can be overwhelming and at times confusing. I want this book to simplify exercise for those who simply want to be healthier. To be honest, most of us just need to move our bodies more.

Some may say the only thing you need to keep fit and healthy is the right attitude, and I could not agree more. The right attitude will steer you down the best pathway for you and your family to help achieve a healthy, fit and fulfilling lifestyle.

I have read many books on health, wellness and keeping fit. I read them because they interest me, and I want to learn as much as possible about my body and how it works. All the books I have read have impressed me in some way; I have taken something from every book, film, and documentary or learning experience I have had in this industry, and even from before I started in the fitness game. Most people in our field have their own opinions about what is needed to keep fit and healthy. I believe there are many ways in which you can achieve health and wellness; no one method is correct or incorrect, and all of them will offer you something.

My philosophy is based on what we call "functional training". This is a form of training that adapts the body to perform activities you would normally do every day. The emphasis is on core activities and building general strength and aerobic capacity without concentrating on any specific discipline. So, "what you need to keep fit and healthy" list is based on the functional fitness principle.

I have already written about the demise of the physical activities we once needed to undertake in the old days. But while few of us now work as hard, physically, as our fathers and their fathers before them, at times we still need to perform tasks we should be capable of, but are out of practice at. Functional training may fill that void.

You really need only three things to help you keep fit and healthy. Motivation, the right attitude and a venue, park or space. Of course, we could add many other things to this list, but the basics are contained within these three areas.

If you go to the gym every weekday for an hour and include a couple of days on muscle strengthening exercises, you are meeting the requirements. How many people do that? You may do CrossFit, yoga, Pilates or boot camp regularly and not only be happy with this but also get more than your recommended exercise needs. Well done! But don't stop reading! I can show you how you can supplement your paid gym or boot camp program with some simple exercises around your house, without being out of pocket. After all, the main thrust of this book is to show you that exercise should not cost a lot of money. If you have the motivation, a good attitude and some appropriate space, exercise is quite literally free.

Let's assume you meet most or all of the recommended exercise requirements. Well done; keep it up. After all, those that maintain their health and fitness are to be commended. If you are one of these people, and you are reading this book, I hope you will also get something out of it. But if you are not meeting the basic requirements, we need to address the reasons why and how I can help you. Those of you who need help, and a reason or motivation to live a healthier life, are more likely to want to keep this book nearby for regular reading and reinforcement.

Simply stating what is needed may not be enough for you. If that were all that was required, I would just ask everyone to read the recommendations. We all respond to different stimuli. The following are some of the reasons I like to include regular exercise in my daily routine:

- I want to maintain my strength for as long as possible.
- I enjoy being able to run, as opposed to enjoying running.
- Regular exercise maintains my general health.
- Playing with my grandchildren is a priority, and I love doing it.
- Travel is so much more enjoyable when I am "travel fit".
- Riding my bike and enjoying the scenery is more enjoyable when fit.
- My resistance to illness increases with good health.
- I love maintaining my hand–eye coordination with brain exercises.
- Regular exercise lets me enjoy great food in moderation.
- A sense of well-being.
- I like how I look. I don't obsess about it, but I don't want to be overweight.
- My clothes fit better when I am slim.
- I enjoy the feeling of not being bloated. I feel lighter when in shape.

- My strength, though reduced by age, is still sufficient for the work I do.
- I maintain my balance.

Some of the above items are similar to those in Dr Kenneth Cooper's list in chapter 1; everyone will have their own reasons for wanting to exercise. The above list is not exclusive, and some reasons may seem a bit superficial, but looking good represents a massive health boost. There are, no doubt, many more direct and indirect advantages of maintaining a regular exercise program. You may have some of your own. If you simply want to look good and exercise helps you achieve that, good for you. Looking good helps your overall confidence and mental health. Feeling and looking good are great motivators, but keep in mind that good overall health is really what we all want, long after our concern about how we look lessens. Looking good and feeling good go hand in hand. If you love looking good, that in itself is a great motivation to keep active.

MOTIVATION

Let's be honest—we like to look nice. Smart clothes and a healthy-looking body would be on most people's list of what this entails, but body image is an individual thing. I don't go for the wafer-thin look, or the extreme image put forward by models, which is obviously unrealistic, but which men and women seem to want to emulate. A safe and sensible BMI is in most instances a reasonable standard to adhere to. I will discuss some other important measurements later on.

A healthy way to think about your body is that you want to be healthy and fit enough to feel good. This is something you can achieve and maintain. Looking like a model in a glossy magazine may not be easy, and we are even told that magazine models can require electronic enhancement to look that good in print.

I know a lot of people who are aware that their diet is not good. They may even know what they have to do to be healthier and fitter. Some make the necessary changes in their lifestyle; some do not. Some say they want to be healthier but do nothing about it. We might say the person who has the right motivation makes the necessary changes. Being motivated is a personal thing. A motivated person might get up at dawn and exercise for an hour before breakfast, then continue with their daily routine. But an unmotivated person may struggle to get out of bed and procrastinate about doing so. You are in the best position to know how your motivation is triggered. An unmotivated exerciser may be very motivated about gardening, or their work or family. Motivation levels vary depending on the task and its urgency. If you find motivation a concern, the following tips may help you become excited about exercise.

Write down your goal or goals and how you intend to achieve them, and include a timeline for completion. Often, writing down your goals makes you think deeply about what you want to achieve. Recording your goals is a great way to think through the process of how you may achieve these goals. It also confirms on paper what you want to achieve and how you intend to do it. This can inspire you and make you more realistic and personally accountable. What you write down can be dynamic; you can adapt it depending on how you approach the execution of your goals. I often readjust my physical goals throughout the year depending on circumstances and what I have achieved. Take some time to think about what you want and how you will achieve it. The thought process is well worth following through. Don't rush this and seek as much information as you can. Research can be inspiring and motivating.

Keep company with people who help, encourage and inspire you. Nothing good will come from being around negative people. They will give every reason under the sun for you not to succeed. Rather, seek out people who encourage and inspire you with their support. You can do whatever you set your mind to, and having positive people around makes the job much easier than having self-doubts brought on to some extent by people who find fault or reasons why you cannot achieve your goal. Look for those in your circle who build you up; this includes family members. I would advise you to sit down and tell your close family members what you want to achieve and request they help you physically and psychologically. Often, if you verbalise your goals, you not only get people including your family on-board, but they may also physically join you in your pursuit of a healthier lifestyle. There is a lot to be said for writing down your goals and keeping the list nearby on a bedside table, your work desk or a note stuck to the fridge.

Plan rewards for achieving mini-goals. Incentives are great to help you maintain motivation. You might save some money for a little holiday, or buy that new bicycle you were after. You may find that it's enough of a reward on the way to weight loss, for example, when you do your weigh-in or measurements and see progress. Whatever the little or big rewards you set yourself, they can help you to work towards reaching your overall goal or mini-goals on the way. You may have a six-month goal to lose weight, run that 5km circuit or lift your own body weight. Your mini-goal may be to reach a certain weight by a particular time, run 3km without stopping or lift half your body weight. I know of someone who likes to have a couple of beers on Friday if he has achieved his weekly goals. His reward is two beers on Friday after work.

Track and record your achievements. This will reinforce your determination to work hard and achieve your goals. Keep in mind that your goal may be a lifelong one; even if you don't have any mini-goals along the way, remember to reward yourself for remaining disciplined and becoming healthier every day. I still keep a diary of my physical achievements and look back on my results with some pride. I am a lot slower, not as strong and my reflexes aren't what they used to be, when compared with myself at 19, but that's to be expected. I get a lot of enjoyment out of looking at my old records and keeping some degree of accountability for myself with my current exercise activities.

Read inspirational books or go and see true life movies. As a boxing enthusiast, I get a lot of personal satisfaction in seeing old boxing matches. Johnny Famechon, Lionel Rose and, of course, my childhood hero Mohammed Ali have all inspired me. I love to see old newsreels and interviews with these champions. I still feel, after watching them that I could go out and become a world champion. I can't, of course, but the feeling I get by watching these boxers and modern local heroes like Jeff Horn, the Australian world boxing champion of 2018, makes me think I can achieve similar heights. It is uplifting and makes me feel good. The feeling is temporary, but it's enough to give me a kick-start in thinking about my health and fitness. Motivation may come and go, and you need to be able to recognise will pick you up, even only temporarily. Some people have told me that watching the Olympic track and field events inspires them to go and run. Some do just that after being inspired by a particular athlete or event.

Be realistic and don't bite off too much. Just start and enjoy small gains. When you think of large goals, they often seem unachievable and too far away. Breaking them down into smaller sections and only concentrating on those can often make a larger goal seem closer. A few years ago, I arranged for a group of my exercisers to walk 96km in 39 hours. The event is called the Kokoda Challenge, and is held on the Gold Coast in honour of the successful but costly military campaign in New Guinea between Australian and Japanese soldiers during World War II. The challenge takes place in very hilly terrain, and some consider it the toughest team endurance event in Australia. We had around 50 walkers and support staff when we started training for this event 10 months out. We started slowly and gradually increased the distances, walking over progressively more mountainous countryside. On the weekend of the event, we had a very successful outcome from a team finisher's point of view. According to the event coordinators, a high percentage of competitors drop out during the event. Of the 24 walkers in our teams, we finished with 21 (87.5%), since three retired due to injury. I have no doubt that one of the biggest reasons for our success was the way we compartmentalised the event into easily manageable sections.

Remind yourself of your goals daily. Kerri Pottharst and Natalie Cook won gold for Australia in beach volleyball at the 2000 Sydney Olympics. Both ladies were interviewed many times after the games, and attributed much of their success to reminding themselves daily of their ultimate athletic goal: to win the gold medal in Sydney. They were almost obsessive about how they focused on and verbally repeated their goals daily. Although just talking and thinking about your goal alone is not enough, it does remind you regularly of why you get up to train and the reason for the intensity in practice. Find ways to remind yourself each day of what you are trying to achieve. Handwritten notes on the fridge, bathroom mirror, bedside table or car dashboard, or in your office, are some suggestions. You could also change the desktop image on your computer so it reminds you of your goals when your computer starts up, or make notes daily in a diary specifically for your aims and achievements.

Tell someone about your goals, or post them on social media, to make yourself more accountable. I must admit, I often think this piece of advice is a double-edged sword. What if you tell someone your goals and you fail to achieve them? Well, that is the point—your desire to avoid that situation can sometimes motivate you to keep on track. Telling someone you trust that you intend to work towards a specific result can also be worthwhile, even if it's just to use this friend as a sounding board. We all need some advice or a sympathetic ear from time to time. The person or people you tell about your goal may well be the one to give that advice or support, and their interest may help you keep on track. This is particularly true for close family members. Telling them your goals may help them understand what you want and how you are going to achieve it.

Don't entertain negative thoughts. This may seem easier to say than to do. Negativity creeps into every part of our life, and it can be hard to change that, but it must be done. I don't mean that you can't think of negative things—of course, we have to be realistic—but, in general, you will benefit from keeping a positive outlook. How you do this will be connected to your personality. I tend to be positive in my outlook on life, and seldom experience long periods of negativity, but I also implement the second suggestion on this list, keeping company with people who help, encourage and inspire me. That helps a great deal. I try only to be around people who maintain a positive outlook on life. These people are gently encouraging without being over the top, but are also realistic in their approach. I have a good friend who I seek out in times of self-doubt and discuss these issues with him. I always get back a sensible response that is realistic but geared towards helping me get out of my slump and back into working towards my goal. If you find negative thoughts are creeping in, don't entertain them longer than you must. Get back to preparing yourself for moving towards your end result. Keep in mind that advice contrary to what you may want to hear may not be negative, but rather realistic. Make sure you differentiate between the two.

Get some help from friends or experts in the field. Often, I feel Australians are reluctant to seek help from professionals. It may cost initially, but often professional advice is just what the doctor ordered. Go and get an exercise program from a personal trainer and chat to a like-minded friend or family member. Keeping your insecurities or concerns to yourself is not ideal. Though we all need to keep our own counsel sometimes, help is also always available, even if you have to pay for it. In my experience, most professionals are great value and well worth their consultation fee.

Don't be discouraged for long. Why "for long"? You will be disheartened at times and feel that you have not reached any of your set goals. Take it on the chin and get started again. Little bumps in the road are inevitable, and you will get down from time to time. It will pass. When all else fails, start again. It is easy to say and write, and not so easy to do, but it is important that you do not stay dejected. Get back into the program as soon as you can. I am reminded of a quote attributed to Terry Goodkind: "If the road is easy, you're likely going the wrong way."

Well, that's my list. It is not exclusive: you may have other ideas about what it takes to keep you motivated and on track. But give my suggestions a try. What can you lose? If you cannot manage all of them along with your own strategies, at least try most of them. You may be surprised at how effective they are.

ATTITUDE

Apart from motivation, I believe you also need the right attitude.

The Cambridge Dictionary defines "attitude" as: "a feeling or opinion about something or someone or a way of behaving that is caused by this". We often hear people say someone has "a terrible attitude" or "a great attitude". Having a great way of looking at things, or a positive opinion about anything, may be described as a good attitude. You will know at least one person who you believe has a good attitude.

In my work, I see good and bad attitudes all the time. The person who is always trying hard, even if they may not always be the most physically capable, is great to be around. You know they may have some self-doubt, but they give it a shot anyway. Conversely, you will know people who may be reluctant to try new things, be that from a lack of confidence or poor attitude. They may refuse to attempt anything outside their comfort zone. It is hard to always be critical of those who seem to exhibit a poor attitude, because we may not know where it comes from, or how their attitude has been formed. The best we can do is attempt to try to encourage them to have a go and see what the outcome will be. Those of you who have made the decision to be healthier, develop a great attitude and adopt a better lifestyle have a greater chance of success.

Poor attitudes can invade your space if you are faced with them regularly. Be aware that attitudes, both good and bad, positive and negative, seep in eventually. You need to guard against being over the top with positivity or, at the other end of the scale, too negative. Both extremes are easily recognisable as being just that—extreme.

I served in the military for over 21 years, and spent nearly a quarter of that time in various positions at the Australian Army Recruit Training Battalion, or 1RTB as it was called then. Daily, I would see recruits that I predicted would make a successful soldier and do well at recruit training simply because of their attitude. Being enthusiastic, keen, alert and willing to learn are all clear indicators of a good attitude. Over a short, but intense period, instructors at 1RTB became very adept at making mental notes on who would be successful and who would struggle. On many occasions, I have trained very good soldiers who cruised through recruit training without too much trouble. However, some of those who seemed to sail through displayed poor attitudes. The Army takes the view that while results are important, displaying the correct attitude is also a highly sought-after characteristic. The significance of skill, intelligence and ability can fade if they are not accompanied by the right attitude. Someone who has the right attitude is often more trainable than someone who does not. If you are untrainable in the Army or in life, it severely curtails your options.

Attitude can be changed for the better. I know this because I have done it in a number of areas. It may be that attitude changes with age, experience or particular incidents that occur during one's life anyway. I have changed my attitude to several things simply because I have a mentor who I respect who points out that we all observe and feel things differently based on our beliefs and genetic character traits. Being more open-minded has helped me to change my attitude about several long-held beliefs, which in turn has helped me be more positive about some issues and to be a better and more positive role model. So don't despair: your attitude can be improved, and your opinions changed.

Develop your mind and train your thoughts to produce a positive attitude to your health and wellness goals and your lifestyle. Your body will thank you for it in so many ways.

Currently, I am training a lady called Nadine, who is keen to join the Australian Defence Force. She is in her fifties and close to the cut-off age for enlistees. The selection process is not easy, and together we have discussed how hard it will be. Ultimately, Nadine may not make the grade, and we must accept that, but we will continue to give our best and do everything possible for her to achieve her goal.

Let's take the worst case and say Nadine doesn't make the grade for whatever reason. We are working hard for her to

meet all the physical requirements, and have talked about how there is no negative side to this. Nadine has become fitter and stronger both physically and mentally, and has become a more confident and positive person in the process. There is no downside.

Last, a piece of advice from my wife, Margaret: "We all have choices in life. You can choose to be happy or unhappy; you can choose your own attitude. It starts when you get up in the morning. Choose to have a good day and start off with the right attitude." Thank you, Margaret. Practise making the right choices.

A PLACE TO EXERCISE

Even prisoners in jail are given an exercise yard, and perhaps a gym and access to weights. I use prison as an example as the importance of maintaining health and wellness may be even greater for those in prison, depending on their circumstances and whether they work while there. Exercise may be a viable outlet for them. You could argue that the lifestyle of a prisoner may be more relaxed than those who are not in prison and you would have a good case. The point to be made is that even those people who have been restricted severely have been given some space and possibly equipment to maintain their health. Whatever your situation, you need space or a venue to exercise.

Sometimes I hear people complain that they cannot afford a gym membership, have nowhere to train or lack equipment to help them become fit. Visiting a gym is great if you can afford it and have the time. Some choose to buy equipment and exercise at home, while others use the services of a personal trainer.

Well done and good for you if one of the above applies. However, money or the lack of it should have no effect on your health and well-being.

Later, I will talk more about incidental exercise, most of which is achieved without spending any money, using objects and equipment that are around us every day. Lack of space can be a hindrance, and it is human nature to want a bit more space, time or different equipment to work on. But we are also clever, and can adapt most exercises to suit our environment.

Lack of space didn't worry Navy Seal Squadron Commander Randy Hetrick, who, on deployment in 1997, developed a system that used a ju-jitsu belt and parachute webbing for a form of body weight exercise called suspension training. According to Hetrick's website, this was the very first version of the TRX strap system that is now sold around the world for use in a highly developed method of exercise. It is particularly useful in small areas.

Innovation and invention come through adversity. You can adapt and overcome most situations if you have the motivation.

CHAPTER FOUR
MY TOP EXERCISES

A debate about the best exercises for you to do would be interesting and lengthy. The powerlifter would have opposing views to the runner, and so on. Generally, it is accepted that *strength*, *stretching*, *balance*, and *aerobic*-type training are the mainstays of keeping fit. I have included exercises from all four of these groups. Sport is also very important, and we make mention of this as well. Not everyone plays sport, particularly as they get older, but everyone that can exercise should, in some form or other.

1. Push-ups
2. Squats
3. Lunges
4. Chin-ups
5. Crunches
6. Walking
7. Running or jogging
8. Swimming
9. Cycling

The above list is a basic pack, if you like. You can add to it or adapt the exercises to suit your likes and physical ability. There are, for example, many variations on the push-up. In fact, I suspect a whole book could be written on the different push-up variations, so there is plenty of scope for you to explore and experiment. If you only did the exercises I have detailed in this book, it would be more than enough. Repetition and effort measurements are mentioned in detail later.

As I have said, any exercise is better than none. However, certain exercises maximise the benefit you get from the time spent doing them. Exercise is good, but specific exercise is better. The exercises are not listed in order of priority. You can select the activities that best suit your needs and resources. Keep in mind that you can do many of these exercises without any special equipment, space or expense.

Before you start any exercise program, you should first check with your doctor. Your doctor is the best person to help you, particularly if you are just starting an exercise program and have not exercised for some time. I suggest you ask for detailed information from your medical professional so that you are aware of exactly what exercises are recommended for you and what exercises should be avoided.

One of the biggest issues I have with some people who have made the decision to commence or recommence exercise is that they overdo it, become injured and dejected, and some-times drop the idea altogether. Others become so excited and inspired that they seldom rest and may become obsessive about exercise. If you do this, it may wear you out over time, and you may leave exercise never to return. Later, I will discuss in more detail how you can resist the attraction of these extremes.

Use caution when beginning a new program of exercise. You will be keen and ready to go, and that's fantastic, but if you are not careful and measured in your approach, you may do yourself some damage and sustain an injury. Take your time initially and be cautious until you feel you are fit enough to increase the intensity. Your body needs to adapt to the additional workload.

This is an exciting time for you, as you're starting out, and I can understand your enthusiasm. Remember that Rome was not built in a day and a steady approach is best. Your confidence, health and fitness will grow together. Let's begin.

STRENGTH TRAINING

Strength training is very important and cannot be ignored. This is particularly true as we get older, when the need to maintain strength may not be as apparent. However, the loss of muscle mass in old age can be drastic. The real importance of strength training is to help maintain strong bones and skeletal structure. You can burn calories and maintain good weight loss with strength training, but strong bones and bone density can be even more important.

Strength training is often called resistance training, and vice versa. Although we immediately think of lifting heavy weights when we think of strength training, there are many more ways to build strength. Of course, in addition to the above, weight or resistance training helps you maintain a firm body shape that indicates you work out, and it can keep you lean, with good posture and skeletal form.

From a functional point of view, strength or resistance training needs to be programmed into your schedule regularly, or as part of your weekly workout. You will come to love the time you allocate to resistance exercise. It helps keep you strong and feeling great. Remember this recommendation from chapter 1: **Do muscle strengthening activities on at least two days each week.**

A few words of caution in relation to strength training. Ego can get in the way of sustainable and consistent training some-times, so regardless of the activity you are doing, be careful to listen to your body. If you are not used to the workload, you will have to condition your body to adjust. You will become sore, and some minor injuries may occur. A sensible approach to your program will see you move through this initial period. Your body will thank you for it! This is often where working with a buddy or mate is helpful. Apart from the obvious safety benefits, a workout buddy can help you maintain motivation and encourage improvement. Injuries can occur particularly if you are not careful and measured in your approach.

Strength training using body weight

The military push-up

Starting position as the photo on the next page depicts. Lower the body to the ground and push back up into the original starting position. The body does not touch the ground but should be just off the surface before pushing back to the orig-inal position. Variations include wider hand position, on the knees and incline push-ups, among others. The push-up with a clap in the middle at the raised position is a social media favourite, but it is an advanced exercise. The push-up is a fantastic body weight exercise.

Feet can be slightly apart to aid balance, and the body should be straight with the head aligned with the body. Great for upper body strength and core stability. The lady in the picture below was one of our clients for many years. Although in her sixties, her form and position for the start of the push-up is excellent and she is clearly in great shape.

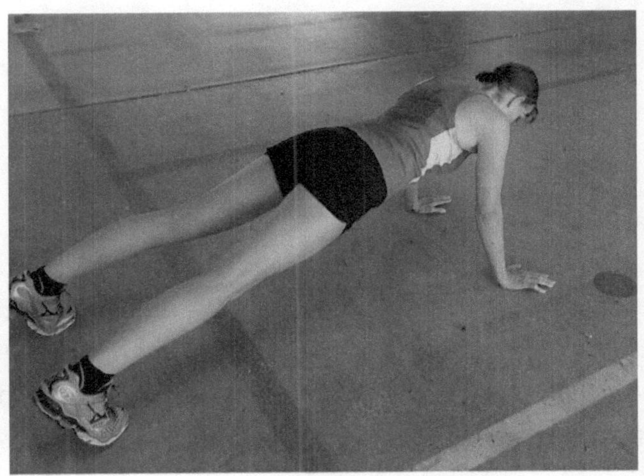

Starting position for a military push-up with feet apart.
Hands directly in line with shoulders. It is important to
ensure the body is straight and the core is engaged to
reduce the chances of the body sagging in the middle.

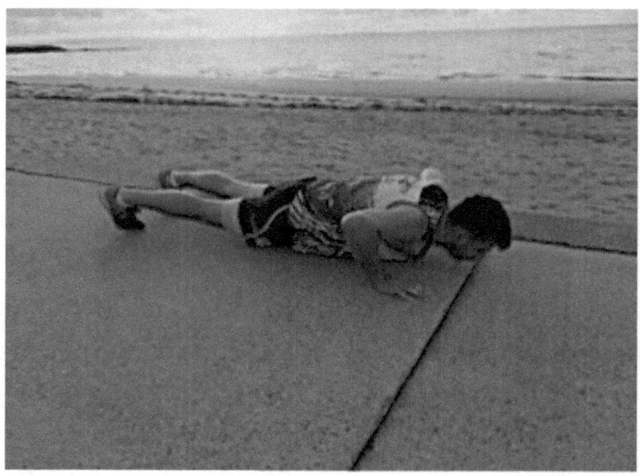

The body should be just off the ground before pushing back to the initial position. Note that the head is in alignment with the body and not sticking up or down.

A military push-up is generally considered to be more beneficial for the triceps, and is often called a triceps push-up. A whole chapter, and perhaps even books could be dedicated to the humble push-up. Without a doubt, it is the most popular and physically effective body weight exercise, and can be done almost anywhere.

The following two photographs show some of the push-up variations, including incline push-ups on a bench and push-ups from the knees. If you have back issues, you may find doing push-ups from the knees much more forgiving. **Push-ups work your pectorals or chest muscles, deltoids or shoulders, triceps, the backs of your arms and the abdominals.**

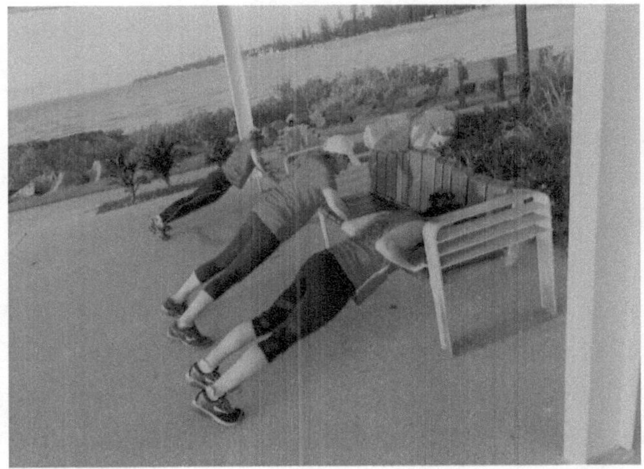

Incline push-ups at a group training session.

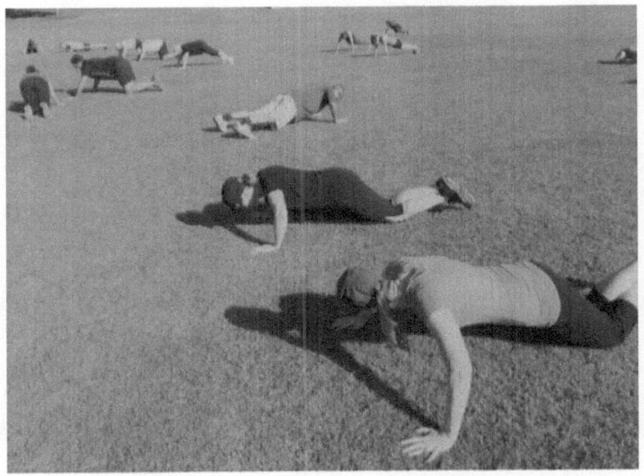

Push-ups from the knees can be more forgiving, and used as a springboard to full push-ups or as an alternative. Common faults with the push-up include: head down towards the ground, a sagging back, and arms too far away from the body.

The squat

The squat also comes in many variations, including using weights. The basic body squat involves nothing more than you and a few feet of space. Put your feet shoulder width apart and bend from the hips, with your bottom moving towards the ground. Arms can be held anywhere, but keeping your back straight and balanced may be easier with your arms forward. Squat as far down as you can and raise yourself back to the starting (standing) position. Try to keep your feet flat and off your toes. Work on not letting the knees move out past the line of your toes.

A squat is a compound exercise; this means it uses major muscle groups and moves multiple joints. The quadriceps, upper leg muscles, lower back, glutes, backside and hamstrings, along with the abdominals, are being activated when you perform squats.

Like most exercises, and certainly the ones I've selected in this book, there are many variations of the squat. A staple body weight exercise, the squat engages major muscle groups and is beneficial from a muscular and skeletal point of view.

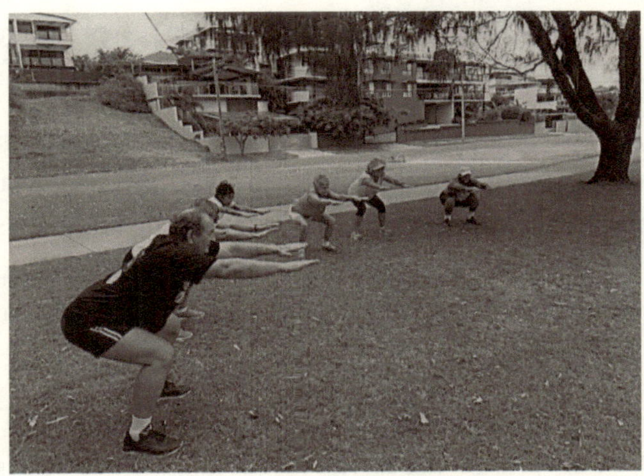

Keeping your back straight and balanced in a squat may
be easier with your arms forward. You can place your
hands on your hips or even behind your head for
variations.

One of our free local government program groups for the
community demonstrates the squat position above. Feet
should be shoulder width apart; bend from the waist with the
feet flat. Make sure the knees do not track over the toes from
the knee in a line down to the foot. You will find that your
weight is transferred on to the heels, so be careful to keep
balanced. The above photo shows the group with arms straight
out from the body. This helps you to remain balanced. You
only have to do a handful of squats before the muscles feel the
extra work, particularly if you are completely new to exercise.

The lunge

The lunge is also a great exercise for major muscles. Standing
upright, you move one leg out, planting it on the ground.
Bend both knees to move to the lunge position, then return to
the starting position. Repeat the same process with the other

leg. You can do mobile lunges, static lunges or lunges with weights.

Lunges are also a compound exercise and benefit the major leg muscles while including the glutes and abdominals. Make sure you keep good form: a straight back with shoulders back. Engage the abdominals to ensure you keep your balance. This exercise is great for improving balance and it also requires good abdominal control.

In mobile lunges, you simply traverse the ground. Do one lunge on the left leg, move up to that leg, then do one lunge on the right leg and so on.

The jumping lunge involves simply jumping with both feet off the ground and transferring legs at the same time. The jump lunge can be very challenging and is considered an advanced exercise.

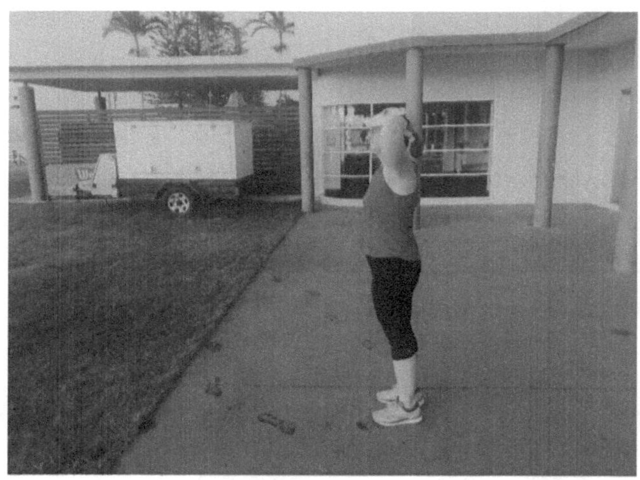

Cathy showing one variation of the lunge with her hands
on her head to aid good posture.

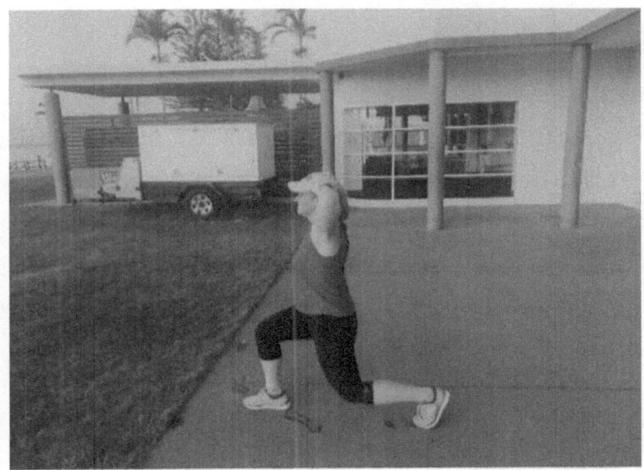

Move one leg out, planting it on the ground, then bend both knees to move to the lunge position. Protect the knee of the trailing leg by ensuring you keep the knee clear of the ground.

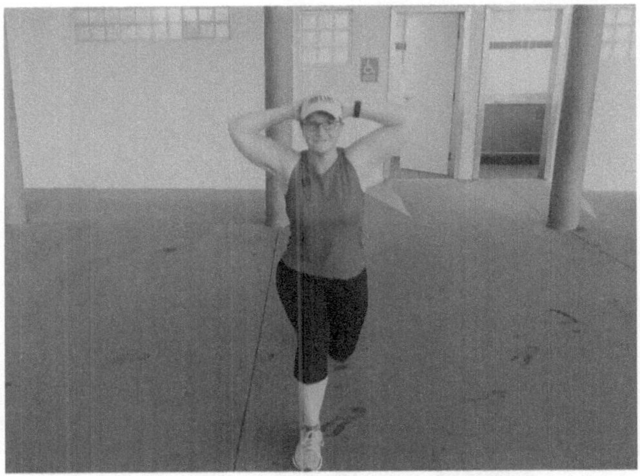

Make sure you keep good form: a straight back with shoulders back. Engage the abdominals to ensure you keep your balance.

Chin-ups and pull-ups

The chin-up is not an easy exercise to achieve, but well worth trying. Chin-ups and pull-ups are terms often used for the same exercise, but technically, chin-ups have the palms facing the body approximately shoulder width apart, while pull-ups have the back of the hands towards the body with a grip position wider than shoulder width. Both exercises work the biceps and back muscles.

Initially, take your time and work slowly rather than explosively.

Other names for these exercises include chins and heaves. What we call push-ups are often referred to as press-ups, for example in Britain.

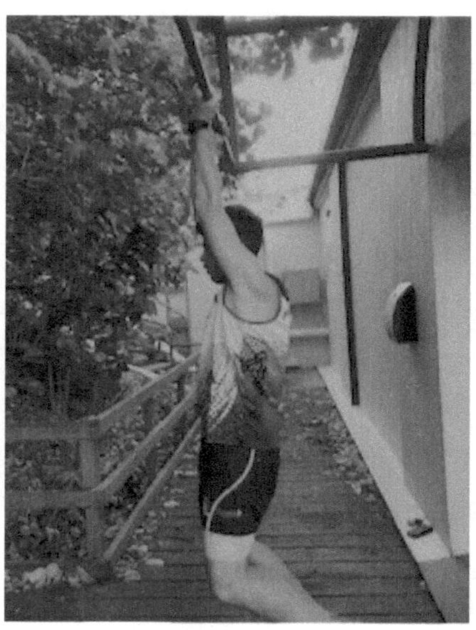

Starting position: arms straight, feet off the ground.

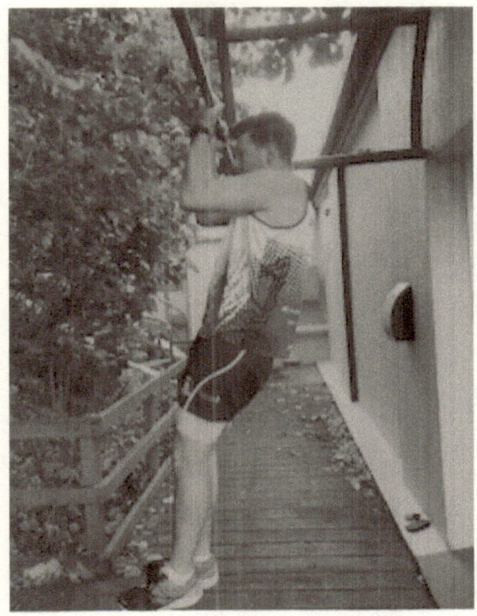

Pull up slowly and with control.

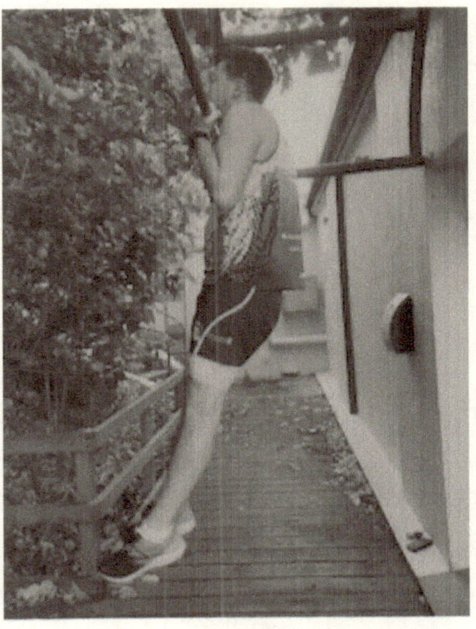

Chin above the bar, pause.

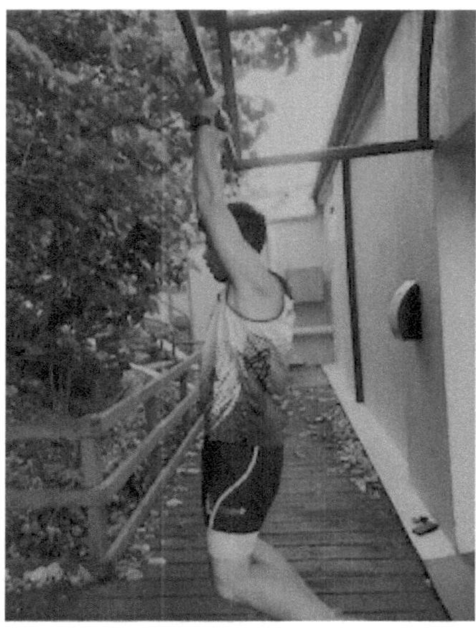

Then lower to starting position.

One of the ways to train to become stronger for the chin-up is to jump up and get your chin above the bar, then slowly lower yourself down. Aids such as straps or a partner assisting can also help you with your chin-ups or pull-ups.

Initially, make sure you can reach the bar and bend your legs to take the full weight of your body. Don't be too hard on yourself if you can't do a chin-up or pull-up. Keep in mind that you are pulling all your weight up to the bar.

Assisted or negative chin-ups are where you use a step or stool to reach the bar, then simply take the weight of your body, slowly lower yourself to the ground and repeat. Chin-ups are great for building strength. The chin-up exercise is challenging but should not be avoided due to its difficulty. Work on technique and keep practising. Because chin-ups and pull-ups also work the muscles of the back, it is possible that you may strain muscles in this area, so be careful and preferably work with a buddy.

The crunch

Hands on the side of the head or ears and back flat against the floor, legs raised. Raise your body off the ground towards your legs and, at the same time, move your legs towards your head and shoulders. Hold this position momentarily and repeat. Resist the urge to jerk and do this quickly. Keep it controlled. Do not lower your legs to the ground until you have completed your required repetitions.

This exercise works the abdominals or core. Use a mat or soft surface for comfort and to avoid back injury. Do not attempt crunches on hard surfaces.

The name crunch is very appropriate. You will agree when you try a few. Of course, if you know and prefer any other abdominal exercises and have done those before, you can substitute your preferred option for the crunch.

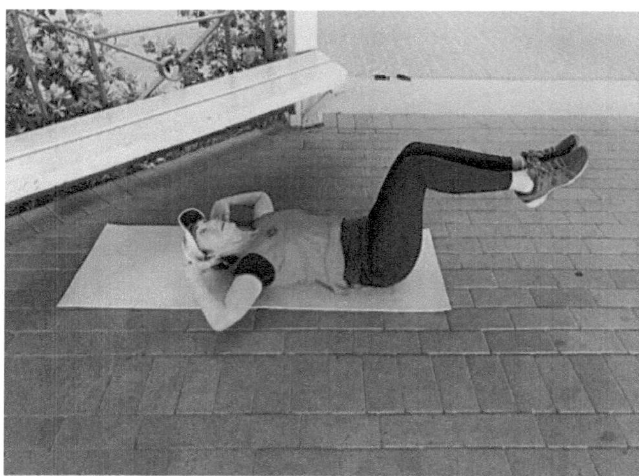

Hands on the side of the head or ears and back flat
against the floor, legs raised.

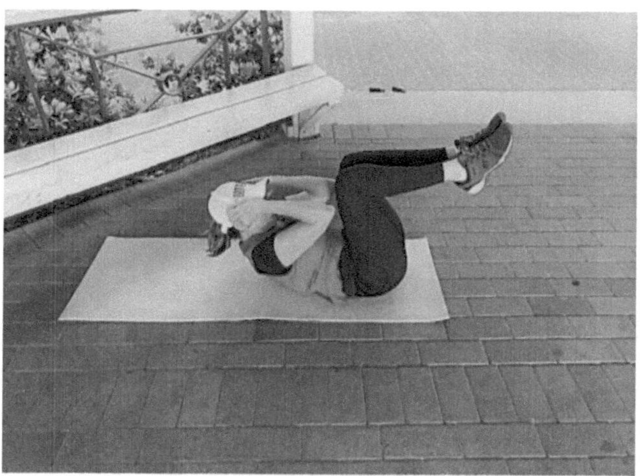

Raise your body off the ground towards your legs and, at
the same time, move your legs towards your head and
shoulders. There are many exercises that target the
abdominals. I believe the crunch is not only a terrific
exercise, but also one that is relatively safe and achievable
for beginners and advanced exercisers alike.

Repetitions of body weight exercises

How many repetitions should you do? It is a good question. The answer will vary depending not only on your strength and capability, but also on the time you have allocated. If you're an elite athlete or budding sports star, your program will be specific and detailed. But for general health and wellness, we don't have to be so accurate. The following are my suggestions on how you can work out your repetitions for body weight exercises.

- Try all the body weight exercises to determine which you can do.
- Do the maximum amount of each exercise you can without stopping. Record this amount.
- Set your subsequent repetitions at 50% to 75% of your maximum in three sets, a set being one round of exercises.

For example, if do ten push-ups before muscle failure and fatigue sets in, set yourself or your program to do between five and seven or eight repetitions of push-ups in three sets (rounds), with at least a 30-second break in between sets.

After some time, you may need to reassess the repetitions of a particular exercise as you adapt and become stronger. Simply go through the process again.

Note: Continue to exercise until your form or posture starts to deteriorate. Basically, that means you become out of shape and start to use your body in ways not intended within a particular exercise. Stop, rest and reset. Then continue. Working with poor form is not only incorrect; you may do damage to your body, and then your program will be affected for some time. Your confidence may be dented, and you may even cease to exercise altogether. Take your time, do the exercise correctly, and stop and rest when fatigue sets in.

If you exercise at home, use a mirror to check you are doing the exercise properly. If you have a partner available ask, them to look at you exercising and help you make any corrections. You can do the same for them.

AEROBIC ACTIVITY

Dr Kenneth Cooper pioneered the aerobics points system, which was based on a person reaching his or her training effect through exercise. That meant their heart rate was high enough to benefit them physically. Dr Cooper believed all people should undertake a minimum of three days of aerobic activity each week, preferably four, with at least one day's rest. Aerobic simply means with oxygen. The process of burning oxygen by exercising and breathing harder is considered aerobic activity in its basic form. Exercises that make us breathe hard and get our heart pumping are considered aerobic-type exercises. The following are examples of aerobic activity. Aerobic activity is a must along with strength training. Basically, aerobic means "using oxygen", and an aerobic activity is one that gets you puffing.

Aerobic activity improves cardiovascular function, and examples include jogging, walking, boxing, football, dance and any exercise that requires you to use oxygen and breathe heavily. The importance of aerobic activity comes from its involving the heart, lungs and vascular system to help transport oxygen to all parts of the body. When we become inactive, our system slows. Like any piece of machinery, we need maintenance to keep us in good working order and particularly for our circulatory system to function properly. Aerobic activity and strength training are two of the main pillars of physical fitness, and therefore good health. Keeping your circulation moving is very important. Our life's blood is exactly that, and you need to keep the highways (arteries and veins) for it open and flowing. Once again, remind yourself of the recommendations: **Accumulate 150 to 300 minutes (2½ to 5 hours) of moderate intensity physical activity or 75 to 150 minutes (1¼ to 2½ hours) of vigorous intensity physical activity, or an equivalent combination of both moderate and vigorous activities, each week.**

WALKING

Walking is one of the best low-impact exercises, if not the best, and is something most of us can do.

Jogging and running are excellent. However, as we age, or if you have had overuse injuries, exercise involving jogging and running may simply not be possible. If you can walk, even slowly with a limp or a walking stick, you can still get some much-needed exercise.

The good thing about walking is the lower impact effect on your body. Months after you were born, you learned to walk, and with some exceptions, barring injury, you will continue to do so until you die. So walking is second nature to nearly all of us. You can walk fast or slow, long distances or short, you can carry extra weight, you can walk as a form of transport or you can simply go for a stroll. You can choose tracks, trails, flat, uphill, downhill or a combination of all these. There are so many variations associated with walking, and for those of you who have no hope of ever running again, it is an ideal way to get some great all-round exercise.

Where I live, I am aware of at least three vibrant walking groups, and I see walking on a regular basis. And it's all for free! Walking can be aerobic depending on the speed at which you walk. The faster you go, the more effort you put in and the more you puff, the more aerobic or cardiovascular your walking is. The actual point at which walking becomes aerobic will depend on many variable factors. What is important is that when you walk for fitness you should do so at a pace that warms your body up; perhaps you perspire and your breathing becomes more rapid. Walking for leisure or transport is still beneficial to the body, but may not necessarily be aerobic.

RUNNING OR JOGGING

Running or jogging gives you the best bang for your buck. Perhaps that's not the best way to put it in a book that is promoting *free* exercise, but you get the idea. Free is the best bang for your buck you can get.

My response to people who ask why I run is generally "because I can". I don't consider myself a good runner, and in the last few years, I have really become a jogger. A generally accepted definition of a jogger is a person who runs slower than a runner. Runners tend to be people who are often out of their comfort zone, whereas joggers may run longer and slower. If you like to run, jog or even shuffle, great. Keep it up as long as you can, because as we age, many of us experience worn out joints and running can become uncomfortable. In many instances, it is no longer possible at all. Running or jogging is a fantastic way to get aerobic exercise, so give it a try while you can. It is good for you.

Like walking, there are many ways running can be varied. You may want to run on trails in bushland, pathways or tracks, up hills or in parks. Short distances, long distances, fun runs, park runs and relay runs, just to name a few, offer further variation.

Many people I know have told me they cannot run, but after some encouragement, they start jogging, even if only for a short distance. Go to one of your local parks and, after doing some warm-ups and stretches, give jogging or running a try. You may be surprised. Having been in the health and wellness business for a long time, I have known many people who told me they just do not run and never want to. I respect that, and understand how they feel. Some of those people who never wanted to run have been gradually introduced to running and now love it. Why not give it a try?

SWIMMING

Swimming is a fantastic low-impact exercise, and benefits the very young and not so young. Use your local pool, the beach, river or dams. Record your progress. Medical practitioners often consider swimming a great form of rehabilitation due to the lower impact effect on the body.

Swimming gives you a great all-round body workout, is fantastic for the arms, core and legs and, because the water provides resistance, you can burn a lot of calories. The buoy-ancy of the water assists those who have arthritis, muscle sore-ness, and aches by giving them some pain relief. While perhaps not always easily accessible to everyone, swimming is a great way to exercise. In Australia, we are lucky that most people live close to water, and we have many public swimming pools. Swimming is almost part of the Australian DNA.

Even if you cannot or do not swim, walking in water provides great low-impact resistance. Treading water may be seen as an exercise for only those doing exercise rehabilitation, but that is not so.

Many people have told me of the therapeutic effects of being in water. Those with musculoskeletal aches and pains particularly appreciate swimming's lower impact on the body. Check out the pools in your area. You may be surprised at how many are available. Some smaller commercial indoor pools may not have the public profile of the larger community facilities, but they can be just as useful. Remember that all the exercises we mention require you to become regular and consistent in your approach, and swimming is no exception.

CYCLING

Cycling, be it stationary or on the road or bikeways, is not only a great form of exercise, it is often used for transport. I mention transport because when I was a lot younger, I don't remember many cycling enthusiasts riding around the streets. A lot of people used bikes to get to and from work. Now, fast-forward 50 years or so and I am convinced the scenario is reversed. Where I live, in Redcliffe, Queensland, we are swamped with racing cyclists whizzing around the streets, mainly on the weekend.

If you are new to bike riding, look for the safer areas and bikeways in your neighbourhood.

Cycling will increase your cardiovascular efficiency, build strength in your legs, improve your coordination and balance, decrease body fat and help increase bone density. Apart from the aerobic benefits of cycling, like walking it can become a good way to enjoy social interaction. The exercise group I am part of plans regular social bike rides around our area.

You can get right into cycling. It can cost a lot of money, or you can buy a cheap but sturdy second-hand bike for transport or exercise. If you haven't been on a bike for some time, start slowly: it may take you a little while to balance and regain your confidence. Use bikeways and safe cycle paths, at least initially. My wife and I have a tandem bike, and we love going out in our local area on it, but my wife prefers me to be leading at the front.

Should you choose cycling as your preferred form of exercise, and you want to buy a bike, go to a bike shop and speak to one of the professionals. There are so many variations of bicycles available, with adapted cranks, high handlebars and even tricycles. Gearing and special additions are available to assist the novice or returning rider.

Bike riding is so much fun and great for fitness. Remember how much fun you had as a child on your bike?

Note: Aerobic activity is not limited to the above. You can, of course, achieve the same effect playing many sports and team games. Sport is mentioned in more detail later.

BALANCE

Maintaining balance becomes more important as we get older, and although we may not practice balance specifically as we age, many of the exercises we have suggested here promote good balance. Squats, lunges and push-ups all help to maintain good balance.

The connection between old age and balance is real. Many in the medical profession believe maintaining balance as we age is vital for good health and well-being. Apart from the obvious advantages of keeping good balance and posture simply to keep your feet beneath you, good balance may have a direct bearing on our health as we age.

Bone density decreases the older we get, and muscle deteriorates. Joints become sore and stiff. Falls as a result of poor balance can cause fractures and other, more serious injuries. Maintaining our balance as long as we can by doing a few simple exercises may stand us in good stead later in life.

Practice at home by standing on one leg for as long as you can. Alternate legs. If you can do this, then try the same exercise with your eyes closed. Join a T'ai Chi class or take up dancing. Practise walking in a straight line. Raise your body up on your toes and maintain your balance for as long as you can.

When we were children, we played many games in the schoolyard and at home that promoted and encouraged good balance. Hopscotch, handstands, headstands and ball games all helped to improve balance. You may not have access to these games anymore, but practising your balance at every opportunity will help you and your long-term health.

The other day, I noticed an elderly gentleman walking along the foreshore boardwalk, and he had his arms out like a tightrope walker while placing one foot in front of the other on the slightly raised boardwalk edge. As I passed him, I said good morning, and he must have sensed my curiosity. "I am practicing my balance," said he. Well done, sir.

STRETCHING

Stretching may not always be included in lists of the best exercises you can do, but it is in mine. In my office, I have a book on stretching. Among all the technical fitness books, including the videos and manuals I have, *The Complete Guide to Stretching* by Christopher M. Norris is the one I reach for the most.

Stretching alone, as a form of exercise, isn't enough, but as an accompaniment to exercise, it is very important. Flexibility helps to maintain good healthy muscle fibres. Flexible muscles help to maintain joints and movement. Shortened muscles, which are seldom stretched, promote bad posture and restrict joint movement. Stretch as often as you can. I include yoga and Pilates as examples of stretching, although that will not always please enthusiasts of these disciplines. Both Pilates and yoga are exceptional exercises to improve core strength, control and balance.

You have been stretching since you were born. Come to think of it, as we get older, we probably stretch much less than we did when we were younger. Stretching, or flexion to use the correct terminology, is very important for several reasons. The basis of most health and wellness programs is movement. If you move less, muscles shorten, and flexibility and range of motion is affected. It is important that body tissues are taken through their full range of motion to maintain their elasticity and extensibility. If this does not occur, the muscle can shorten and, in some cases, that shortening may become permanent.

Shortened muscles can cause pain by applying pressure on the bones and joints of the body. It is important that we maintain our flexibility for as long as possible to maintain good posture and a full range of movement.

In this book, I only scratch the surface in regard to stretching. Much has been written on the subject, and the ability to stretch and keep your flexibility for as long as possible will stand you in good stead as you age.

In an ideal world, we would stretch before and after exercise. Although there are many theories around the importance of stretching and its execution, there are a couple of basic principles.

First, before stretching, warm up your body with a fast walk, slow jog or stationary cycling, star jumps or jumping jacks. This has the effect of increasing your heart rate (pulse), which in turn pumps more blood to the body and muscles. Your rate of breathing increases and your body starts to prepare physically and physiologically for exercise.

Depending on what you are going to do, concentrate your stretching on the major muscle groups for that exercise. For example, if you are going for a walk, a calf, hamstring and quad muscle stretch would be most appropriate. If you are going to work your upper body with body weight exercises, then arm, torso and upper body stretches will be more relevant. Hold the stretch for about 20–30 seconds and ensure you feel the stretch, but no pain. A longer period of gentle stretching is preferable to shorter, more dynamic stretching. Take some time after strenuous activity to cool down and stretch the muscles used during the exercise session.

Once again, be aware of your body and any restrictions you may have in relation to stretching. Start off doing some easy stretches. Try to stretch every day. Consistency in all forms of exercise is very important. Yoga is an excellent discipline for stretching and keeping the body flexible. A few people I have known have never attended a group yoga session, preferring to practise in front of the television in the comfort of their own home. This is another example of the opportunities we have to keep our bodies flexible, in good shape and healthy.

It is generally recommended that you hold each stretch for approximately 20–30 seconds, as mentioned above. Stretching for longer may not provide any additional benefit; it is up to the individual. A good habit to get into is to stretch whenever you can: at your desk, during your lunch break and whenever you have a few minutes.

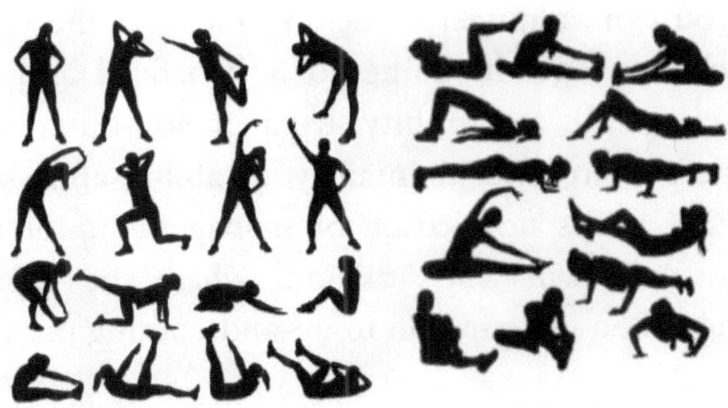

Some stretching and body-weight exercise poses.

As I mentioned before, you can adapt the exercises to suit you. You may not be able to do lunges, but find squats are fine. Just remove lunges from the list. If you cannot do squats and lunges for whatever reason, that is okay. You may put more emphasis on swimming or walking, for example. The exercises can be made simpler if need be, or made more difficult by adding weights, doing more repetitions or working slightly longer. It is up to you.

A FEW WORDS ON SPORTS

Sports play a big part in many of our lives, and in our health and wellness, even at an advanced age. I recently watched a YouTube video of a person running in the 100m sprint in the United States. That person was 100 years old. I played Masters Soccer and had a few games in the over 35 and over 45 categories last year. Of course, we're not going to set the world on fire with our speed and ability as we age, but we can still participate at a competitive level in golf, tennis, squash, touch football, netball, table tennis and the list goes on.

If you feel you cannot now participate in the sport you love, perhaps you can volunteer to be an official at the very least. The exercise you get in doing so is beneficial and you are giving back to the community. It can help you in so many ways to keep sharp and maintain your ability and skill level. Some of my mates now coach or manage a junior sporting team. This is a win–win situation, where the experienced coach can pass on information to up-and-coming players.

Some people play sport once a week, and perhaps train once or twice a week. Sport can play a big part in people's overall health and wellness, provided it is consistent and regular. The type of sport you play has a big bearing on your health and wellness. Pool or snooker and darts, while considered sports, may not have the same beneficial overall health benefits of playing tennis, squash or handball for example.

So, there it is: my list of the only exercises you need to do. You may need a good pair of gym or running shoes, a top, shorts or pants, and bathers if you include swimming. No other expense is necessary.

Of course, if you want you can buy a cap, water bottle or sunscreen, and the list goes on, but the *necessary* equipment for you to exercise is basic. All the above exercises can be done in or around your own home or local park. Of course, you can do more by adding to the list of exercises if you want to, or if you have specific requirements. The whole point is that keeping fit and being healthy should not be expensive. In fact, many people keep in great shape and never go to a gym or spend money on expensive exercise equipment. I hope, after reading this book, you will join them.

I have seen people who exercise wearing the latest gear, the most expensive shoes and well-known brand name clothing. On the other side of the coin, I see very fit people who wear the basics. Don't get caught up in the marketing spin that you have to have the world's best clothing and footwear. Simple but comfortable is just as effective. The choice is yours.

So, if you have the right attitude, are motivated, have the space and follow the suggested exercises, you are well on the way to becoming a fitter person. You can do this simply, all for the cost of buying this book, perhaps a pair of gym or running shoes, some sports shorts and a singlet or T-shirt. The rest is up to you.

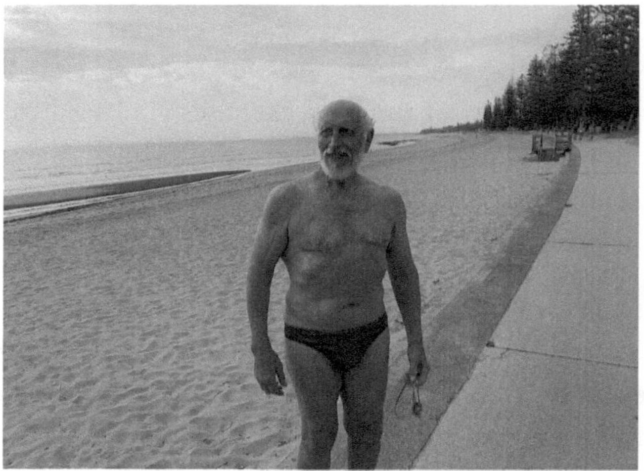

Horrie (Howard Clark, pictured) swims every day of the year at Suttons Beach, Redcliffe, Australia. He is 78 and an inspiration to all who come across him. Horrie was a top sportsman as a youth, and played football at a professional level in his native Wales and in Australia. Horrie prefers swimming daily, with a visit to his local gym, to keep healthy and fit. Over the years, he has had at least two instances I know of where he has been badly stung by jellyfish in the water. One of the toughest and fittest men I know.

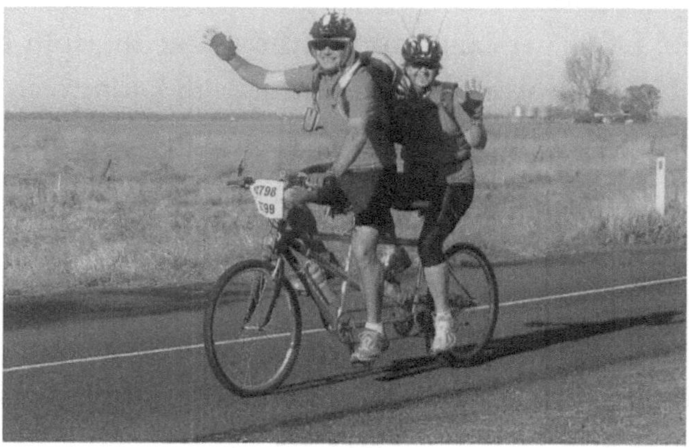

My wife, Margaret, and I riding in the Queensland countryside on our tandem bike.

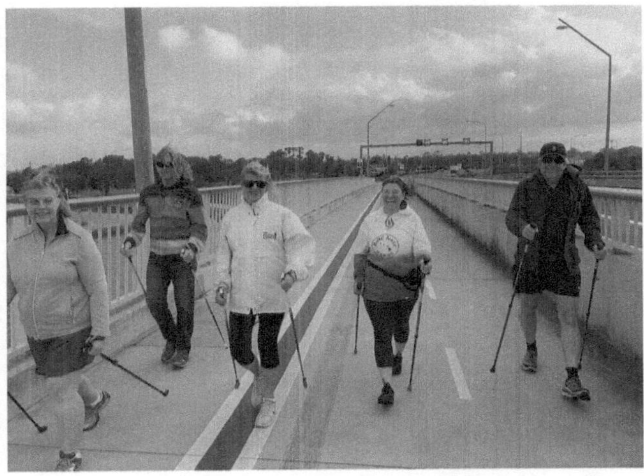

A local Nordic walking group out on a blustery,
invigorating day.

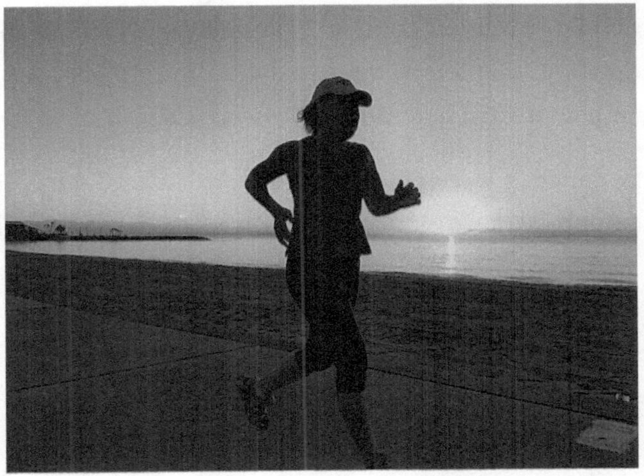

Kenna runs along the sand at Suttons Beach just before
sunrise.

Should you have problems executing any of the exercises I
have detailed in this chapter, simply take them off your list. As
I mentioned before, you can adapt the exercises to suit you.
You may not be able to do lunges, but that is fine. Just remove

lunges from the list. If you cannot do squats and lunges for whatever reason, that is okay. You may put more emphasis on swimming or walking, for example. The exercises can be made simpler if need be, or made more difficult by adding weights, doing more repetitions or working slightly longer. It is up to you. Work out what you can do and write yourself a program

Read what Marjorie has to say about her exercise group that meets weekly at no cost.

Tom is an inspirational exercise guru

We first met Tom when a group of people showed up at Thurecht Park, Scarborough, Queensland, for Moreton Bay Council's Healthy & Fitness free program in 2018. Tom showed us the best exercises for balance, bone strength, coordination, physical strength and even touched on exercises for our cognitive functioning.

As the council's weekly program came to an end, we decided as a group to keep going without a personal trainer. Five months later, a group of us is still meeting at the same time at the park to continue exercising with the knowledge and support Tom had given us. Tom showed us, and told us many times, that you don't need expensive equipment or to join a gym to keep fit. As well as using the machines in the park, we do a series of warm-up exercises, stretching and cardio. Tom has said many times, "it's not that you can't do that exercise you once did as a young child, it's because you just don't do it anymore." He suggested that anyone can start exercising at any age. Now, after all these weeks, what can I say about a man who so graciously still gives up his time to visit our group, inspire us with new exercises and information … and what's on about the traps!

Thank you, Tom.

Our exercise group is a pure example of how free exercise can be achieved.

MARJORIE SMITH, SCARBOROUGH
EXERCISE TEAM

WHERE, WHEN AND HOW TO START EXERCISING

If told you I could reduce your chances of falling ill and contracting diabetes, while helping you sleep better, improving your appetite, giving you more energy and making you more alert, you'd jump at the opportunity, wouldn't you? The surprising thing about all the above is that most people can achieve it all for free, but many don't because you need to jump in wholeheartedly.

Let's look at where, when and how you exercise. It might all sound a bit easy, but taking a few minutes to sort this out is worth it. Any time spent planning your exercise will benefit you down the track, and can boost your interest and enthusiasm in your program. Even if you're not big on planning, sit down, take some time to look at the best way for you to get your exercise program in, and when and where you will do it.

WHERE TO EXERCISE

You can exercise just about anywhere.

Over the years, I have had several taxi drivers attend my classes. I devised a program for one of the drivers to get his stretching done in the cab and at the kerbside during down-time. He could easily do this incidental exercise when waiting for jobs at the taxi rank.

A group that exercised with me in a boot camp setting made a point of stopping work before morning tea, getting together in a circle and doing some gentle exercises before making a cup of tea or having their break. The time allocated was additional to the break, and their employer was happy to give them some time to exercise daily. No doubt there were additional benefits to the office staff gathering for ten minutes to exercise, including the chance to have some work-related conversations. It was a great way to fulfil a couple of requirements in one go. I am told that the team loved it, and why not?

One of our larger general goods retailers in Queensland has allocated a set of exercises to be completed voluntarily and daily by its employees. The business even referred to the exercises using funny and quirky names, staying away from what some see as the technical jargon some trainers and those in the fitness industry use. These exercises were done in the staff lunchroom.

Another who attended my sessions told me he influenced his boss to have the staff meetings while riding bikes on stationary trainers. A bit noisy, I would imagine, but interesting and unusual—it would have been a lot of fun.

I have been invited to present healthy activities to the staff of a local hospital on a regular basis during their lunch hour. A number of the staff have devised a program of activities and healthy option presentations as a team, working within Queensland Health, and were awarded a certificate of excellence by their superiors for having the foresight to produce and implement the program. A makeshift gym was quickly arranged in one of the hospital's conference rooms, which proved a great initiative. I have to say that those who attended had a good or even high level of overall fitness.

A local radio station I was lucky enough to visit gives its announcers the choice of sitting down or standing up to complete their shift. Standing while working is much better than sitting, we have learned, and some announcers choose to stand and present.

If you travel a lot and your job has you staying at hotels, you may have access to a gym or park. I am not sure of the percentages, but based on my limited knowledge and personal experience, I would think that hotel gyms are not all that well attended. If this is true, I wonder why people do not use facilities that are free and provided for them. It amazes me.

Cruise ships are sometimes considered to be basically floating hotels. These ships seem to have a good attendance history at their gyms. Though this may defy my assumptions about land-based hotels, I have a theory about why this is so. Those who use hotels for accommodation and work often have tight schedules and timelines due to business pressures. Their leisure time may be limited, and some people, while away from home, use every minute they can being productive for their job. So the time they have to use the gym, even though it's free, may be limited. Let's take the luxury cruise ship gym for a comparison. Aside from staff, the thousands of people on-board are all having a holiday, their time is their own and the atmosphere is relaxed. So there is time to go to the gym. Add to that, the food on most ocean liners is amazing and plentiful, and the gym provides a fantastic counter to the increased calorie intake. Or is it just wishful thinking on my part that cruisegoers would look at it this way?

The list of examples above is my way of saying that you can find somewhere to exercise regardless of your situation. Don't use lack of space as an excuse. Of course, there may be limitations and restrictions, but I would prefer we see them as challenges, not reasons to not exercise. I have heard people say they have nowhere to exercise. Is this just making an excuse? If you have space to sit or stand, you have room to exercise. It may be limited, but the space or place where you do your exercise can be adapted to suit your needs, and you can utilise the available area. In an ideal world, we would all have access to any facility we desire, but until that happens, we need to adapt and use our imagination.

WHEN TO EXERCISE

Now is the best time to exercise. I do mean that. Put this book down, get up and go for a walk; you can come back to it.

My point is, don't procrastinate, and don't overthink exercise. Just do it. As one of the famous sporting company slogans points out, "the longer we wait or analyse, we tend to find reasons against any positive thoughts we might have." Just do it now.

Let me be a bit more practical. The best time to work out is the best time for you. It has been my experience that if you get a group of people together, you will almost always find a difference of opinion on what may be the right time to exercise. Some, and I would suggest maybe even most people, do not have the option of choosing their preferred time to exercise. In an increasingly time poor world, many simply exercise when time permits. I would think this is true of most of the working world.

In the morning, the body has effectively run out of carbohydrates or sugars for fuel, and it switches to burning fats instead. One way that it does this is by releasing a substance that "turns on" the fat cells to release their fats. Because of this, some people believe it is better for fat loss if you exercise in the morning. You can find many examples and studies that suggest that morning exercise is better for you. Journalist Mimi Spencer reports that "sports scientists at Glasgow University have found that, while morning exercise may feel harder for some people, it can be a great mood booster, setting you up mentally for the day."[1]

Getting up early can help boost your physical energy and mental alertness for the day ahead. I must admit, afternoon exercisers seem more likely than early morning exercisers to not turn up due to work commitments, bad traffic and so on. My experience supports the improved mood theory; it certainly seems to hold for my early morning clients.

Over the years, I have had many contracts to work with corporate clients in or near their work environment at the end of the working day. I can tell you, my experience with this time allocation is not as good, and nor is it as well received as is my work with clients before starting work in the morning.

For some time, I worked with a couple of schools to provide exercise for their staff at the end of the school day, and once again, I was often confronted with absenteeism, lethargy and overtired teachers. Many excuses were offered regarding poor attendance. Some of the excuses may have been convenient, but, nonetheless, attendances were affected. I also believe that many people are not in the right head space for exercise at the end of the day. They may be tired and worn out. On the other hand, some people much prefer to work out after work and have no problem with afternoon or evening exercise.

Afternoon classes and some evening classes may be harder to fill due to people having had a full day and being tired. Sometimes exercise takes a back seat. Of course, some people do not leave work on time, or may encounter traffic problems, bad weather or overtime. All these reasons can affect people getting to afternoon or evening classes.

My personal preference is for morning exercise; luckily, as an exercise professional, I believe I work best in the morning, though I try hard to be consistent all day as required. Mornings and early mornings are my preference. It is fair to say that I have also been conditioned to exercising in the morning.

Incidentally, the Tom's Law 5am Wednesday session is the second-best attended morning session I run. A bit early, you may think, but it does give people plenty of time to get home, go through their morning routine and get off to work on time. Numbers are naturally affected in the cooler months, and you may find you are not keen to exercise in the early morning in cold weather. It is a personal decision.

Mid-morning sessions are very popular with young mums and senior citizens. I am not excluding men, but my programs, and others I observe locally, are heavily attended by ladies. This makes sense. Some fitness professionals and gyms specifically program mid-morning activities to cater for mums who have dropped children at school or who may have a pre-schooler in tow. A lot of gyms and private operators now provide child minding services to allow busy young mums to get some exercise in. While my focus in this book is not gyms and paid exercise, if you have small children, you will have to consider them in your overall exercise plan. I see plenty of people exercising in our local area running with prams, squatting with babies and even using small children as weights. Once again, you will need to adapt based on your own circumstances.

For over five years, I ran a free community exercise program that started at 9am. It was almost exclusively attended by senior citizen women. Being a free program, it was ideal for those on pensions or who had stopped full-time work and had the time during the week for a 9am exercise session. Many attendees would walk, play golf or ride bikes at other times. They were a great example of the people in the community who pay very little, or nothing, to exercise. Their combination of great experience and thrifty thinking is a very good example to highlight. The social aspects of exercise were also very important for this group. Remember that the women I describe above were mostly retired or on a pension of sorts. They not only did not want to spend a portion of their pension on exercise or gyms, but also needed to keep a close eye on their daily finances. I understand that and agree with their choice of a free way to exercise.

Lunchtime is a very popular time to exercise for some office workers and those who travel long distances, or for a long time, to get to work. Such people use the time they have available. They are often time poor, but rather than not get any exercise at all, they use their lunch break to stretch their legs, go for a run or do whatever they can in the time allotted. Lunch, like any other time, has its advantages and limitations for exercise. The heat may be a factor in some countries. Does your work have showers and changing facilities? When do you get to have your lunch if you take the time to exercise? And the questions go on.

If you are travelling early in the morning and don't get home until late, lunchtime offers a great alternative to early morning or evening exercise. Just use some common sense regarding the conditions and location. Once again, your daily routine will dictate when and how you participate in exercise.

Over the years, I have had several personal training clients who worked odd or extended hours. I would often schedule their training session for them after they had finished work. One client and her husband could only exercise after she had returned home from working in the city and her young family had consumed their evening meal and been put to bed. This couple exercised with me at 8pm in the evening. Another client and I sometimes found ourselves running at 9pm, after he had finished work, in preparation for a fun run. Now, you can of course do the same for free, but keep your safety and security in mind. I always tell my clients to buddy up with someone if they are doing sessions themselves in the early hours of the morning or at night.

In one of the polls I conducted with people who follow me on social media or get my email newsletter, I found almost a 50/50 split between those who attended morning or evening classes, with the evening winning slightly. This is a small data sample, but it does highlight that opinions are just about evenly divided in relation to morning and evening exercise. I have had a lot of people exercise with me over the years, and although some have left, quite a few remain on my newsletter database. From time to time, I get some useful information from these people, even if the information is different to the experience of my own attendees.

Take some time to plan your program daily and weekly. Make a schedule and ensure you prioritise your exercise so it is completed.

HOW TO EXERCISE

Those of us in the health and wellness industry may take for granted what we do and how we do it. I am reminded of this regularly when people approach me to start up an exercise program for them, and they really know very little about healthy eating and exercise. Although Google and many other sources of information are available, surprisingly, not everyone takes advantage of these information highways. They may not have any inclination to do so. As we also know, Google is a great tool, but contributors to the websites it indexes, along with social media, are not always accurate or their information based completely on science.

How to exercise and how to start exercising are two different topics. I will cover them briefly here. How to exercise is not difficult if you follow chapter 4 and choose some of the activities I recommend. I refer again to the Australian Government

Department of Health, which **recommends exercising by being active on most, preferably all days every week, doing 2½ to 5 hours of moderate intensity activity including vigorous activity, and doing muscle strengthening activities on at least two days each week.** This gives you plenty of options from which to choose your preferred method. Whatever exercises you choose to include in your weekly program, you certainly have plenty of variety. I have highlighted some examples of a weekly exercise program in this chapter.

How to begin exercising is easy once you have decided it is time to start. Arnold Schwarzenegger, of *Pumping Iron* and many other films, is reported to follow a very strict regime of getting up early and riding his bike to the gym every day. Apparently, he does not think about it too much. It is simply routine. Thinking about exercise for too long takes time, and time is important. So often it is better to just get on with it. Getting up and just doing it is easy if you make sure you have plenty of sleep. Allow time in the morning to exercise before heading off to the office or work.

I know people who tell me they have no time at all to exercise because they are too busy. That excuse doesn't impress me. Making a living is important; we all know that. Think about this. If you don't have your health, the percentages tell us that your chances of living a long and productive life may be affected. That may get you started. I know of quite a few people who have been told they would suffer severe health issues unless they started exercising to look after their health. That worked for them.

Start slowly. If you want to run a marathon, remember to be patient. You need your body to adapt to the additional workload. You cannot go from zero activity to flat out and not expect your body to reject it. Be patient, take it easy and do some research. Read about and study the ways in which you can go forward and improve your health. I tell people who have not exercised recently to begin with walking. Do it as often as you can. Once you have adjusted to daily exercise, introduce a little jogging. If you cannot jog, keep walking and adjust your pace and distance. If you can, try jogging the distance between lamp posts. Then, each week gradually increase it to two lamp posts, then three and so on.

The same approach can be taken with almost any exercise program. Start slowly, light and easy, then gradually increase and move towards faster, heavier and more difficult. Consistency is the key to exercise. You must be consistent and regular. You cannot bank exercise; it is a lifelong activity and should be routine, like brushing your teeth. I often have people who exercise with me tell me that whenever they have had a break from exercise and come back to a workout routine, it is hard, and they must work to return to their previous fitness level. Some studies suggest that as little as three days of no exercise or inactivity can affect your hard-gained fitness level. I think it is much easier to get into a healthy routine of regular exercise than it is to regain fitness after a break. Once you have a base level of fitness, you can always adjust and increase your workload for any goal or challenge you have set.

Several things can work against you and your goal of becoming healthier and fitter. Don't let them stop you! The weather, depending on where you live, can be a deterrent. Generally, you need to be aware of conditions in your area and dress accordingly. Your workload, family commitments, social life and general bumps in the road may also hamper your exercise program. These are unavoidable and will affect everyone. Just accept them as they come. Get back into your regular exercise program as soon as possible. It is all about the balance in your life. Become balanced and make your exercise program a priority and part of your daily routine.

Partner up with someone who has similar goals to you. I have a few people in my exercise group who walk or run with one another when they are not involved in exercising with me. These partnerships are so productive and build more than good health habits and exercise routines; often the partners become great mates. There are several instances within the exercise groups where these partnerships include sharing holidays together regularly. Having a partner also helps keep you both accountable, in a very gentle and encouraging way. I have no doubt that a training buddy or partner can become a life-long friend. The variety and type of exercises you do together will vary as time goes on and your ability and goals shift.

Day	Sport	Distance		Start time	Finish time	No. of hours	Sleep	Comments
		Planned	Actual					
Sunday	Swim Bike Run Other							
Monday	Swim Bike Run Other							
Tuesday	Swim Bike Run Other							
Wednesday	Swim Bike Run Other							
Thursday	Swim Bike Run Other							
Friday	Swim Bike Run Other							
Saturday	Swim Bike Run Other							
Totals								

Simple daily exercise program or log (template).

The above is a very simple example of a weekly exercise log. There are many variations to such logs, including weekly and monthly charts. You may want to make up your own. Another column can be used for resistance training activities. You can buy a logbook or use a notepad. When I look back at my log, I find comments like "Not 100% today but did a slow 2km jog," "Fastest 5km I have done since 2004," and "Sore shoulder so still no push-ups for two weeks."

Some people keep a log religiously; others do it to remind themselves what they have done for the week, like keeping a diary. You may want to set out your weekly program on Sunday, for example, and use your diary as a means of keeping yourself honest. Once you have written down your program, you simply must follow it.

I conduct a running group every Friday for an hour. The attendees run or walk distances from 2km up to 7km. I time the attendees and keep their records for them. Now and then, one will ask me for their fastest time, and I just check my records. Most of you will find keeping a diary a good thing to track your progress. It is particularly useful when starting to exercise, and can be a confidence builder. I do also know of some people who have never logged their exercise and are still good regular exercisers. It is up to you. Assuming you want to log your exercise, I have filled in a sample log below from Sunday to Wednesday.

Day	Sport	Distance		Start time	Finish time	No. of hours	Sleep	Comments
		Planned	Actual					
Sunday	Swim							
	Bike	2km	2km	7am	8am	60min	7h	Very windy today
	Run							
	Other	50 push-ups, 30 crunches, 50 lunges						
Monday	Swim							
	Bike							
	Run	Walk 5km		5pm	6pm	60min	8h	
	Other	10 chin-ups and 100 squats						
Tuesday	Swim	20 × 50m laps		6am	7am	6min		Heated lap pool
	Bike							
	Run	2km	2km	6am	6.30am	30min	7h	
	Other	30 × 3 lots of crunches. 10 pull-ups in three sets						
Wednesday	Swim							
	Bike							
	Run	2km run	2km	6am	6.30am	30min	7h	
	Other	50 push-ups, 50 lunges, 50 squats						
Totals		Bike 2km, walked 5km, ran 2km, swim 1km				3h30m	>7h sleep	A good week of exercise

Simple daily exercise program or log (example).

I have mentioned China a few times in this book already. I remember being very impressed when I was there several years ago with my then employer to buy equipment for our gym back in Australia. We travelled to Hong Kong, then caught the train to Guangzhou where world-renowned trade fairs are held annually. I was amazed at the free local facilities in the parks, available to everyone, dotted around the city. Across the road from our hotel was a very large public park and, although it cost a few yuan to get into, the park facilities were amazing. If you wanted to, once there you could stay all day at no extra cost.

Permanent table tennis stations, various monkey bar constructions, fixed badminton nets, swings and sit-up stations were positioned around the park. You could hire electric or paddle boats to use in the large lake in the centre of the park. Government-paid instructors took morning classes in tai chi, meditation and yoga. The park was full of people running around exercise tracks, joining in on group exercises and doing their own morning exercise routines. Okay, Guangzhou is the third-largest city in China, and the place is busy all the time. However, I have never seen people in any other country exercising in numbers anything like what we witnessed in China. I was impressed. To see older men and women demonstrating their flexibility, strength and dedication to being healthy each day was inspiring and, as an Australian, a little embarrassing.

CHECK OUT THE FREE FACILITIES IN YOUR AREA

Most councils list the facilities they have available for public use on their websites or in pamphlets. Where I live, in Queensland, it is hard to travel more than a couple of kilometres in towns without encountering a park with exercise facilities. Most of the equipment is suitable for body weight exercises, with a variety of bars and planks for sit-ups, step-ups and so on. Some of these facilities have full explanations of the exercises and how to use them. Some don't, but then, you don't have to be a Rhodes Scholar to work it out.

You may be well and truly already aware of these facilities or, as some people tell me, they were completely unaware of such structures in their neighbourhood. Where I currently live, there are three separate free exercise areas within 1km, not to mention numerous parks. Do you have any close to you?

For several years, our local council ran a program where fitness providers were engaged to go to fitness stations on a regular basis to show locals, and whoever wanted to turn up, how to use the facilities. I was involved in some of these sessions, and they were very successful. Although there are fitness stations near where we live, they are not always fully utilised. But they are very useful, and are truly appreciated by the people who take the time to use them. David Peters is one who appreciates the exercise equipment:

> My name is David Peters and I have become part of a group that meets once a week. The group was part of an exercise program that was led by Tom, focusing on exercise and movement. Anyone could participate as it is for people of all ages. We still meet at a park in Scarborough, which has an exercise station that we use to do a weight circuit. ... It's fun because of the social part but, best of all, it's absolutely free.

Almost every piece of equipment or structure you see as you go about your daily business presents an opportunity to exercise. I am not suggesting that you spend your day seeking out structures to use to do some push-ups, for example, but if you adapt the way you look at things, opportunities will leap out at you. In the next chapter, I mention parkour, and how the people who love this form of exercise embrace the possibilities of almost every structure they come across. Common sense should prevail: when you use public structures, ensure you are not breaking the law or being dangerous or reckless.

The Moreton Bay Regional Council is the local authority that looks after the area where I live, and it has recently contracted me to conduct some exercise programs. It has allocated the park and equipment to be used, and I've visited the park to check out the equipment. The structures the council have installed there include some body weight machines and one pedal machine with a resistance knob to adjust to suit the fitness level of the person using the equipment. It is fantastic.

I have come across a number of local and state authorities that run free programs for the general public. These free sessions are not necessarily run all year round. Because the budgets are generally quite small, there may not be a lot of advertising done. I would advise you to contact your local council or check out their website to see what they may provide. Certainly, most councils in Australia run free programs from time to time. In my own area, the council organises both free and subsidised programs. Check them out.

Some organisations hold "come and try" days. They are generally free and afford the club running the programs an opportunity to show the general public what it does and how it goes about its business. In my local area, there are several clubs offering activities from dragon boating to martial arts that conduct such free programs. Veterans' programs, assistance for people with a disability, and free programs for the public can generally be found on the relevant local or state government websites. You may need to dig a little, but you will find these programs. If all else fails, call the organisation and ask if they do "come and try" days.

Near where my wife and I live, there is a very well-maintained local park. The grass is always green and well mowed, and there are running lanes around the park and tracks set up for distances from 100m to 400m. Many groups use the park, including one of the schools next door and the local Little Athletics organisation. The local government authority makes sure this park is particularly well-maintained, as it is used by quite a few groups on a weekly or even daily basis. I have seen cricket matches played here as well. Although the park is well used, it is still vacant a lot of the time. Locals use it to get in a few laps, test out their latest kite or drone, or simply take the dog for a walk. Many of us are spoiled for choice, and this is the case where we live. Perhaps your local parks are not as well-maintained or not so local, but by doing a little bit of research, I am sure you will find plenty of exercise opportunities near your home.

I should mention that I have used free government exercise facilities in at least ten different countries, and while location, quantity and geography change, the facilities are generally all the same.

When was the last time you used your local park? Some parks have running tracks on them, but even if yours doesn't, it is a free area for you to exercise. Ask your local authority for a map and locations of the free parks and exercise equipment near you. Get out and into the fresh air and do some exercise. It can be random or structured. You have access to these facilities; it is a shame if you don't use them.

A lady who I have known for quite a few years is known locally as Snodge. I know her real name, but she prefers this nickname. Read what Snodge thinks about the area where she lives and exercises:

> Exercise must be enjoyable! It is necessary for our general well-being. We have so many options available here on the Redcliffe Peninsula, with free outside equipment and activities to suit all levels of ability and taste. Our council is very supportive of the personal trainers and the maintenance of the equipment and parks.
>
> Retirement can be very isolating and lonely. However, I am fortunate to be surrounded by so many wonderful healthy motivated people, including my 80-year old, bike-riding, body-building housemate and the early morning horse

trainers who are at the stables seven days a week from 4.30am in all weather conditions. I also enjoy the company and energy of a group of people who meet and exercise regularly at the "lagoon".

Inspirational trainers can be found along the foreshore with so many activities on offer, including circuits, Pilates, boxing and meta-fit to name just a few. The benefits are many. Strength, flexibility, mobility, energy, good sleep patterns, bone density and, hopefully, weight control and friendship.

Exercise is empowering, enabling good mental health by contributing to a focused and positive attitude, as Snodge explains. What a positive approach to life!

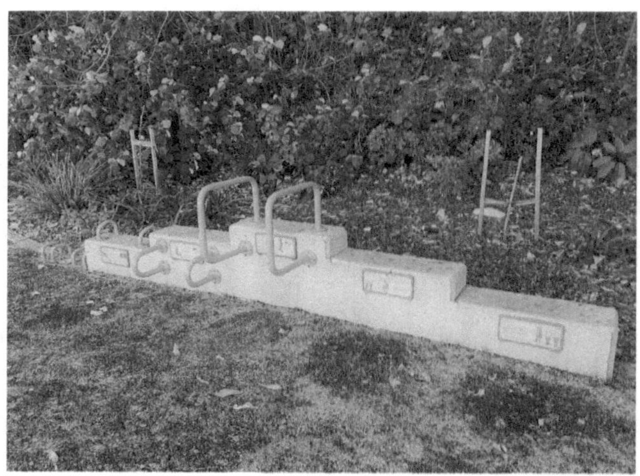

Local free exercise equipment at the beach.

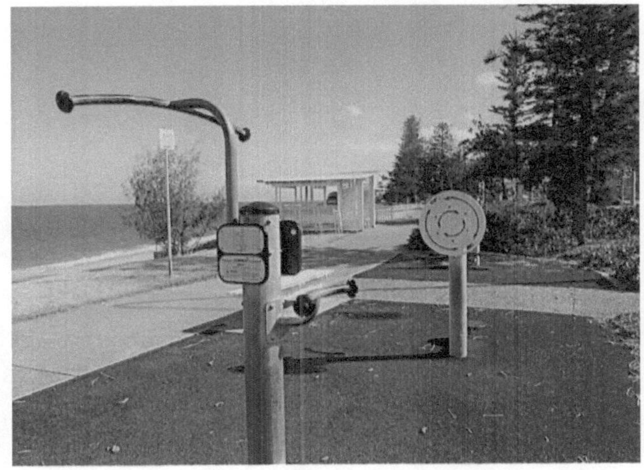

Council-maintained exercise stations along the shoreline.

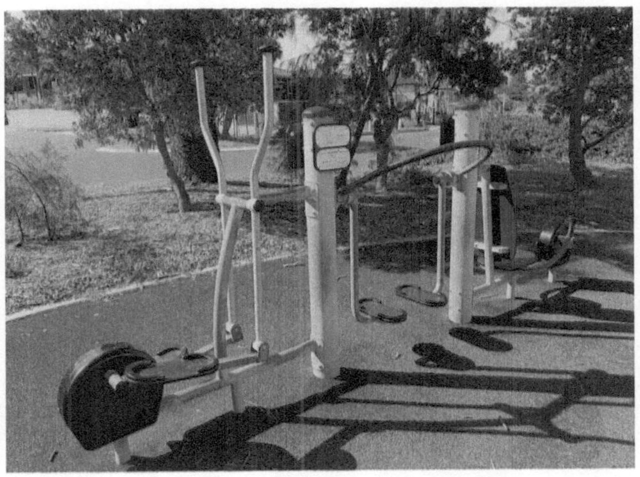

Some well-placed community exercise equipment.

Incidental exercise is the exercise you get during your daily routine, from the moment you get out of bed until you get back into bed. From the minute you get up, you are accumulating incidental exercise and burning calories.

There are plenty of examples where people accumulate a lot of incidental exercise because of the nature of their jobs or careers. Miners, nurses, mothers of young children, school children, outdoor workers, labourers, farmers and wait staff, just to name a few, all get substantial incidental exercise on a daily basis. No doubt there are many more occupations that provide plenty of incidental exercise. Unfortunately, many more people simply do not get anywhere near enough incidental exercise, daily, weekly or throughout the year. The benefits of exercise cannot be banked. We need to approach our health and its maintenance like brushing our teeth. It must be done consistently, ideally every day.

The modern world has given us many devices and machinery

that not only make life a lot easier, but encourage us to live a more sedentary lifestyle. Here are some examples:

- The motor car has given us the ability to travel long distances quickly, and we get a lot more completed in our day. Sometimes, though, we use our vehicle to take short trips that we may have walked in days gone by. Those who were not fortunate enough to have a car often walked or cycled to do daily tasks or to get to and from work. The physical exertion required to achieve that kept our bodies moving, and exercise was had simply by walking or cycling from place to place.
- People who worked in construction or on roads often had to use a pick and shovel to dig holes or trenches. These tasks have now generally been taken over by digging machines or excavators and the physical aspects, certainly in larger projects, have diminished considerably. I am not against progress by any stretch of the imagination. We can now build much faster, repair quicker and make a lot more people safer than we could previously. But in the process, we have contributed to the physical decline of many people.

So, the exercise we used to get as part of everyday life may no longer be available to many of us due to progress. This doesn't apply to everyone, because a lot of people still work hard physically. But the truth is that many more of us now lead lives that include sedentary jobs with a much-reduced opportunity to work our bodies. Add to this the way that we have streamlined many tasks and can do so much more in a day, which leads to us often being asked to perform more duties, making our working day longer and more stressful. Not everyone is in this position, but it represents a fair proportion of our working force currently.

The gym explosion in modern society is due largely to people's need to incorporate a gym session into their daily routine on top of their employment because, in many cases, their occupation no longer provides the activity levels the body requires. In fact, some case studies have concluded that simply going to the gym for an hour and working out on an almost daily basis, may not provide enough movement and activity to compensate for an eight-or ten-hour workday of relative inactivity. That is concerning.

A hundred years or so ago, gymnasiums were used by athletes, gymnasts and boxers, and only catered for those who dedicated at least part of their life to one of these disciplines. Today, 24-hour gymnasiums are so abundant that the competition for membership has made joining a gym easy and affordable. Affordable, however, is relative to your situation. Although I can afford to belong to a gym, my preference is to work out in the great outdoors. One of the aims of this book is to convince you to return to some form of incidental exercise and to program regular daily activity. If you are content in your routine that includes a gym membership, well done. Keep it up!

My wish is that this book will help the reader, to adapt and maintain health, wellness and fitness by making some simple daily routine changes, which in many cases will be completely free. The changes you will see in your body and general outlook are well worth it.

Nothing in life is easy. We all have choices to make. If you choose to change your lifestyle to incorporate daily exercise without paying a lot of money, you will be able to do so quite easily— take it from me. You will save money in two ways. First, you will spend little or nothing on getting and keeping healthier and fitter. Second, you will likely spend less on illness and health-related issues.

WALK MORE

We are so used to having the convenience of a car that we have forgotten one of the best ways to get around is on foot. We get to our destination faster by vehicle, but we miss out on so much more. When we walk, we get the chance to talk to our neighbours and locals around the area. We can also appreciate the nature around us; we take in the weather and, if the sun is shining, we soak up vitamin D.

I walk as much as I can. I live just 1km away from our local shops and newsagent and, although I have driven my car to the shopping centre from time to time, I mainly walk.

Trust me when I say that you will come to enjoy walking. You can dawdle and think about any issue you may have. Often, by the end of a walk, you will have solved any problems in the time you've had to mull them over. Set a great pace and time your walk while working up a sweat, or set a pace that leaves you breathless. The choices are yours. The benefits of walking are many, even from a purely exercise point of view. You will get your circulation moving, and stretch while maintaining muscle bulk and bone density. Walking is low-impact, so it will not aggravate existing trouble with ankle, knee or hip joints. It makes you feel good. Compared to driving, your senses are heightened when you walk: you see, smell and hear many more things.

If you choose, you can walk with added weight. You can carry a day pack with essentials. You can walk for fitness by going faster, or simply walk for enjoyment. Those of you who can incorporate walking into the routine of your working day should investigate how to go about that. You might already take the train to work, maybe getting a bus from the train station to your place of employment. You may even take the car to the train station or get dropped off there. With a little bit of planning and some more time, you could walk to the station in the morning and walk from your destination station to work. The extra time is worth it if you are prepared to adjust. If you must get up 15 or 20 minutes earlier in the morning to fit in the walks and perhaps catch an earlier train, do so. The opportunity for you to be healthier is available, and the choice is up to you. The only cost involved is your time.

One of my current clients does a lot of bushwalking. She not only enjoys the benefits of exercise and all that walking physically brings, but also finds it a great way to de-stress. Walking in the bush and simply getting back to nature helps to calm us, and is so therapeutic for many. You may be able to relate to this. Stress relief is a great way to help clear the mind and refocus.

Walk to the shop to get your paper. Take the dog for a walk. Have your evening meal a little earlier and go for a walk before retiring for the night. Use part of your lunch break to take in a walk around where you work. Not only will it be good for you physically, it may be a terrific stress reliever. Take a notebook and pen with you to jot down notes. Sometimes a walk during the day unlocks many issues you may have been mulling over. Write down the answers as they come to you on your walk. Look at your day and plan where you can walk instead of being sedentary or driving your car. The possibilities are endless and depend on your mobility, determination and the time you spend planning. Give walking a try and stick at it. You may be surprised to see that your lifestyle adjusts and walking becomes habitual.

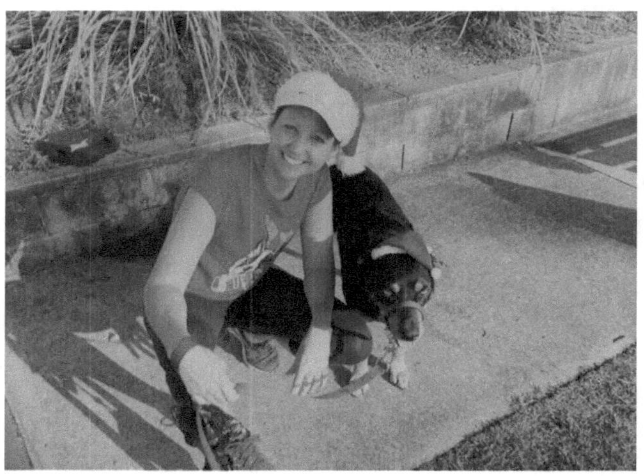

Leeanne exercises by walking her trusty companion Bob.

RIDE A BIKE

It may not be practical for you to ride to work. If so, try cycling to the train or bus station, or part of the way to work. In a share-ride situation I know of, a person rides his bike to his mates' place Monday to Friday, then shares a ride with them into the city. Perfect! This person gets two bike rides a day, five days a week.

I provided a physical fitness test for a very fit gentleman ten or so years ago. He had never set foot inside a gym, played no regular sport and only did compulsory sport as a child at school. His physical fitness questionnaire stated that he did no physical fitness or sports activity at all, yet his VO_2 max score was very high, indicating he was in good shape. After a bit of probing, I found out he cycled to work five days a week, a daily distance of 20km return. So, this gentleman was riding his bike around 100km plus each working week. Apart from a bit of gardening, that was the extent of his physical workout. The reason for his great VO_2 max score was because, although he considered his bike riding cheap transport rather than exercise, doing it five days a week kept him in great shape.

You can pick up a cheap bike that suits recreational riding. Better still, use the bike to get the bread, milk and paper, to visit friends and just to enjoy the great outdoors. Those of us who live in a climate with fantastic weather should take advantage of the conditions and get out a bit more. Bikes provide great exercise, are cheap, don't pollute the environment and are an ideal form of transport. You may have bike paths or lanes in your area. Some cities and towns have purpose-built pathways for pedestrians and bikes. If you are not confident riding in traffic, use the allocated bikeway. Remember, when you ride a bike, you are helping to keep a car off the road, and that can only be good for the environment.

I could go on about bikes, but this is the last word from me. Riding a bike takes a bit of coordination and balance. Those who ride bikes, and have done so for some time, do not realise this, as it is second nature to them, but it is true. Riding a bike is a confidence thing. The longer you can continue to ride safely, the better it is for you. Your confidence and coordination improve, not to mention the physical benefits. Make sure you wear all the appropriate safety equipment required. In Australia, as I write this, it is mandatory for cyclists to wear an approved helmet and to have working front and rear lights when in darkness.

TAKE THE STAIRS

There is a rule in my family that where stairs are provided, we take them instead of elevators, escalators and travelators. If you could see my wife and I at any airport, you may be amused, as we seem at times to be the only ones using stairs. Meanwhile, the escalators are full. It is a simple thing to do: just decide, whenever you can, to take the stairs. Stairs provide a great cardio workout, activating most of the muscles in the legs. This burns a lot of calories and builds muscle. As you would expect, walking upstairs gets your pulse racing and blood pumping around the body much faster. All of us, at some time, have taken a break to get our breath back when climbing stairs.

If you have stairs at work, use them. You could incorporate stairs as part of your resting routine at work. Rather than going for a coffee, go up and down the stairs to get your blood circulating. This will also work out any stiffness you may have from sitting for a time. I used to work at a place that had only one additional floor above the ground level. The stairs seemed to be used only by delivery drivers, because there was always a traffic jam of people waiting for the one lift at either floor. I often passed this group to take the adjacent stairs, smiling to myself and knowing I would be back at my workstation long before the lift people arrived.

Some time ago, in my weekly newsletter for my exercise group, I wrote about a gym not far from me. It was located one floor up in a shopping centre. Alongside the stairwell to the gym was a lift, which I often saw gym users taking up and down. It seemed a little bit strange for people who want to exercise to miss a great opportunity to get in some incidental exercise on the way to the gym.

Some high-rise apartments and office blocks have prohibited the use of the stairs and made them for emergency use only. If this is not the case where you work, try using the stairs more. People tell me one of the reasons they don't use the stairs is because they are slower. While this may be true, I do not believe it always is, as my tale above shows. In the units (apartments) where I live, you can use the lift or the stairs. My wife and I always use the stairs where we can, whereas most people I know avoid them, and miss out on a perfect opportunity to get in some incidental exercise.

STAYING FIT ON A CRUISE HOLIDAY

Many of my clients, like myself, love to go on a cruise for their holidays. We are lucky, where we live, to have a cruise terminal in Brisbane. Departure from there can take you on a cruise for a minimum of three days up to several weeks. Anyone who has been on a cruise ship raves about the amount and quality of food available. The food is a highlight in many cases. After all, you have paid to enjoy yourself, and you should. The amazing variety of well-presented food is fantastic, and many people take advantage of it. If you're concerned about coming home from a cruise a good bit heavier than when you left, you might benefit from my advice.

First, at all costs avoid the all-day buffet meals. The food is so tempting and available that you could not be blamed for spending a lot of time in the buffet area. Stay away! Take the time to go to the dining rooms provided, where the meals are measured and very well presented. It is not as easy to overeat, though you will be given plenty of variety and quantity. You may have to go to your cabin and change from your bathers to be properly dressed for a meal in the dining room, but it is worth it. Of course, you may want to sample the buffet once or twice, but the temptation to go back time and again can be too much. Before you realise it, you have overeaten. The reason the buffet may not be a great idea is it is hard to measure how much you have eaten. Often, when beautiful food is so plentiful and readily available, we eat to excess rather than to satisfaction. There is a whole chapter in this book on food and nutrition, and I am sure it will open your eyes about food consumption.

At every opportunity, take the stairs while on a cruise. Some of the bigger cruise ships have up to 13 or 14 decks. All the cruises I have been on provide lifts. As I see it, these are for those in wheelchairs or with mobility issues. Thank goodness the lifts are available for them. But if you are able bodied, use the stairs.

While I was writing this book, my wife and I visited our daughter, son-in-law and grandchildren in Bahrain. On the way there from Brisbane, we stopped for a short time in Dubai. At every opportunity in each location, my wife and I used the stairs. In Dubai, perhaps one of the biggest airports in the world, we looked very strange. As the travellers piled on to escalators, we cut lonely figures climbing the stairs. **Here is a perfect chance for you to make a conscious decision to do**

one thing today to benefit your health. If you can, and are capable of doing so, from this moment on always take the stairs. Make it a rule.

Last, even if you are not a gym person, go to the ship's gym for 30 minutes or so each day. After all, it doesn't cost you anything. You already paid for it when you settled your fare. Use the walking tracks around the decks; most modern ocean liners have these. Develop a routine of going for walks after meals or getting in a short gym session each day.

The three suggestions I have given you will not in any way, impede your holiday. They could make you enjoy it even more. Would you believe I lose a few pounds each time I take a cruise? Although I work in the health and wellness industry, I put this down to having just three regular meals a day and being free to work out. While at home, I may concentrate on working my clients hard, but on-board a ship, I have the time to do my own workouts daily. You can do the same. Of course, you want to relax and have a great time, but with no work pressures and limited contact with the outside world, you have plenty of spare time to get in a few laps of the exercise deck or 30 minutes a day in the gym.

A few words on alcohol. I enjoy a drink from time to time and, like most people, think it is nice to enjoy alcohol in a celebratory setting. On a cruise ship, there are many bars and the temptation to drink is strong. In fact, it is encouraged. Keeping in mind you are on holiday and you want to enjoy yourself, I would suggest you do just that. Like everything and everybody, we all have our limits. You just need to know yours and act accordingly.

So, there is my advice to those of you who like to cruise, but also like to keep fit and keep your waistline from expanding.

GO DANCING

A good mate of mine, also a personal trainer, runs dancing classes with his wife in our local area. I classify dancing as incidental exercise, because I imagine many people dance for fun. However, the benefits from a fitness point of view are often understated. Dancing requires coordination, flexibility and teamwork, just to mention a few of the necessary capabilities. The aerobic exercise involved in dancing can be very beneficial to your health. Of course, there are enormous social and recreational aspects that you enjoy when you join a dancing group as well. Most local communities have dancing classes at no cost or a very low cost. A few dollars spent on dancing may give you many hours of enjoyment and improve your health drastically. Those who dance often say they prefer to get their workout from dancing over any other discipline. Often, when you are having fun, you may not notice the physical aspects of an activity.

SOME MORE WAYS TO GET DAILY INCIDENTAL EXERCISE

Go shopping or window shopping? The amount of walking you do when shopping may surprise you. People often report that when doing something enjoyable like shopping, they don't notice the exercise at the time. Perhaps later, a sense of tiredness overcomes the shopper, but in the meantime, they have done a lot of walking.

Carry your own shopping. Sometimes I see people wheeling shopping trolleys to their car with only a few items in the trolley. Take the opportunity to use your muscles, and if you only have a few items, carry them. A little bit of weight training will do you a lot of good.

If you use public transport, stand instead of sitting if you can. Make sure you are balanced and stable. Even if the trip is only short, you will be using your abdominal muscles to keep yourself upright and straight. Practise engaging your core muscles while doing this and enjoy a mini workout at the same time. Concentrate on good posture. If you have been sitting most of the day, your body may appreciate standing and stretching its muscles.

Stretch when you can: in the lift, in the car or at your desk. Make a point of getting up from your desk regularly to walk to the water cooler. Take the stairs and stretch. Take five and move your body. Incorporate your walk with a glass of water at the coffee station.

As an incentive, **count your daily steps**. Buy a cheap pedometer or use the step counter on your smartwatch to track how many steps you take during the day. Challenge yourself to doing a regular number of daily steps. Don't become caught up in the accuracy of the device you choose to use to count your steps: use it as a comparative measure to record your steps for added incentive and interest. Ask those in your workplace if they want to do the same and take up the challenge to count steps daily or weekly. One of the groups I worked with for a number of years, gave every one of their staff a Fitbit exercise monitor so they could manage their exercise daily. What a great idea!

Park your vehicle some distance away from the shopping

centre entrance. You know what I mean. If all the spare parks are a short distance from the entrance to the mall, don't do laps around the centre looking to get a closer spot. Why put yourself through the stress? Take the space some distance away and walk to the mall or shops.

Try to arrange stand-up meetings at work. If you stand, you are burning more calories and using your major muscles and core to help you stay upright. People who stand tend to spend less time talking than those who sit, so this may also help to reduce the length of meetings. That, surely, cannot be a bad thing.

If you take public transport, walk to the next bus stop and get off one station back from your normal stop. Walk the extra distance. It may take a little longer, but you get the benefit of some more incidental exercise in your day.

I know a family who refused to buy an electric or petrol lawnmower. Instead, they **use an old push-pull lawnmower.** Some of you may not even know what I am talking about. If you ever get the chance to use one, you will know that it takes a fair bit of physical effort to push it around a lawn, and even more effort and skill to get it to cut the grass.

The last example I want to give you is quite extreme. You will get the idea. Many years ago, some good friends of ours wanted to put in a pool. They had the money and the necessary space in the backyard, but access was a problem. That is, access for machinery to excavate the space for the pool. Rather than be deterred, our good friend and his two boys dug the pool by hand. The pool, from memory, was nearly 2m deep at one end and around 1m at the other end. It was 5m square. Can you imagine how long it took them to dig the hole by hand? It was practical and cheaper, and the father and his two boys saw it as a team building opportunity. More importantly, they made the time. What a story to pass on to your children and grandchildren! I did say at the start this was an extreme case, but necessity and ingenuity worked for them.

I know you will come up with more instances where you can accumulate a lot of incidental exercise during the day. If you look at your day as an opportunity for you to get some exercise, I am sure you will be able to get plenty.

Don't find excuses to avoid exercise. It could be that we are not as fit and healthy as we could be for this exact reason. Many of us spend our days trying to find an easy way to do things, when perhaps we should embrace any opportunity to move our bodies, if it does not affect efficiency. The more incidental exercise we do, the less time we need to look and pay for opportunities to exercise. The money you spend on a gym membership might be put towards your next cruise or holiday, or who knows what?

CHAPTER EIGHT
FREE EXERCISE PROGRAMS
AND THE IMPORTANCE
OF REST

I met Tom whilst walking on the beach and joined a free ladies exercise group, which was a subsidiary of one of his Tom's Law groups. I say find a group you enjoy and walk as much as you can. Enjoy every day. It starts the day off in a beautiful positive way and sets you up with energy for the day. My husband has diabetes and has kept it at bay by walking half an hour, twice a day, in the beauty of the morning and evening.

CARMEL FLETT

Exercise may require a bit of effort on your part, but only a little bit. We all know people who exercise on the beach or at the park. They may even run or walk. Perhaps they can be seen in local parks doing abdominal exercises and body weight sessions. Good on them. I would think that you know of some people who are fit and healthy but have never paid for exercise and don't ever intend to. If you are already like that, well done!

You are already reaping the benefits that consistent regular exercise can bring. Perhaps if you are like the people I have mentioned above, you may already have tried some of the following suggestions.

GET A GROUP TOGETHER

Join with like-minded people through your local walking group, Heart Health or shopping centre walkers, or start your own group of walkers and exercisers with your own friends. Get a regular routine going. Don't be deterred by weather or negative situations. Plough on through. Motivate your family for regular walks on the weekend.

YOGA

Do it at home for free; use an app or follow television programs. Buy a book on yoga and meditation, and learn how to relax, stretch and calm your mind. Self-help books like the one you are currently reading are still very popular for those who want to study and learn in the comfort of their own homes.

APPS

Check out the free apps on your phone. There are literally hundreds of free workouts you can follow simply by down-loading the relevant app. From building abdominals of steel to yoga, run trackers to heart rate scales, there are many free apps. Check them out.

TELEVISION

People in my own family have used the television to enjoy their daily workout. There are still plenty of shows you can tune into to work up a sweat, all free of charge. All you need is some space, time and sensible exercise clothing. Keep a water bottle and towel nearby, and you are set.

COMMUTE

We might be crossing over into incidental exercises, but it is true you can exercise on your way to work. Why not? You may ride a bike to work, walk all or part of the way, or perhaps combine transport modes. Park, walk and ride to work using your car, your legs and public transport. For many people, a daily commute is the best time to get in some regular exercise, as it simply means allowing a few more minutes in your routine. When you get to work, try to use the stairs if they are an option.

YOUTUBE

YouTube is an amazing resource for exercises, often with detailed explanations and plenty of variety. You can find just about any form of exercise there. I find it a great resource for my exercise programs. Like all available information, some on YouTube is good, and some is not so good. Be particular; after a little while, you will be able to sort the good stuff from the rest. Use YouTube as a useful resource, not as sole reference.

LOCAL GOVERNMENT PROGRAMS

I mention local government programs several times in this book because they are a great way of exercising and a lot of local government agencies provide them. You need to simply check out your council website for times and places. I also suggest you give your local government office a call. Even though most now have comprehensive websites, they all still seem to maintain a good call centre. The thing to remember about government agencies is that while they often have programs and facilities available, their promotion of these may be lacking. It always pays to ask them. You may be surprised at what is available, often for free.

PARKRUN

Parkrun is another free event that involves a 5km run, and is conducted around the world. You have to commit to helping now and then, but the program is completely free, extremely popular and very social. I highly recommend Parkrun as it caters for all fitness levels from beginner to Olympian, and the events generally take place in pleasant surroundings, near parks and gardens. A bonus is that your time is recorded. You can get the entire family involved in this activity.

Read a real account of Parkrun from Sheila, a lady who has exercised with me in our free community group. Sheila has a fantastic story:

> In 2013, I was a 54-year-old lady who was fully focused on my stressful full-time job, and had never been into exercise in

any form. I was then diagnosed with a serious medical condition which required immediate surgery. This threw my life into complete turmoil and led me to retire early and to have to re-evaluate my life priorities. As a result of the condition and the subsequent operations, I felt I had aged so much, both physically and mentally. I needed to promote my healthy living options, but with a much-reduced income. What could I do?

One day, in the local paper, the *Redcliffe Herald*, I saw an advertisement for a free exercise group being held on the local beachfront. It was only once a week, but I felt too old and out of condition to take something like that on. I walked past the exercise group on a couple of occasions and noticed it was a mixed age group of people of differing capabilities, but what struck me was the laughter. Everyone seemed to be enjoying themselves. The third time I walked past, I had the courage to approach the group leader about the exercise class being held.

To say that moment changed my life would be an understatement. I joined the class for their once a week session. I then became aware of a local free 5km Parkrun held every Saturday morning at Sandgate seafront. I have now completed a total of 160 Park runs around Australia, and a couple in the UK. A total distance covered of over 800km! I still find this astounding.

From these groups I have met a lot of like-minded people of similar capabilities, but one lady in particular I meet two to three times a week at 6am in the morning to run 5km on a route of our choosing. Having this person in my life gives me enormous motivation.

I have recently become aware of the "Live Life Get Active" free camps in my area, provided by the local council, which I have attended when I get a chance.

I can now say that, as a result of these exercise initiatives I have taken on-board, I have lost weight, improved my posture, gained confidence, made some amazing friends, and truly feel so much more alive and healthier. As I reflect on my journey over the last five years, I realise that it has all been achieved at no monetary cost whatsoever—how amazing is that!

SHEILA MAGNIER RMHN, RGN (RETD)

UNIT OR APARTMENT GYM

There are many apartments or units where we live. On more than one occasion, I have been asked to develop a program for the residents of some units, to use in their on-site gym. It is easy to do and costs very little. I suspect a lot more people living in units would use their gym more if they knew what they were doing. Speak to your body corporate; after all, if you own the apartment, you are a part owner of the gym. You may as well use it.

WALK OR RUN YOUR LOCAL TRACK

Many parks worldwide have walking and running tracks, and you can take yourself there any time to get in some free exercise. Take the baby for a walk in the pram, walk or run with the kids, or take a ball and have some free fun and exercise.

Check out your local newspaper or free monthly magazines

and local government publications. Look on the internet or, as it seems a lot of people do on social media, ask for advice about free classes. Where I live, I am aware of a number of sessions that are being run free of charge. These programs are funded by government or private companies, and some larger property development companies pay health providers to program regular exercise sessions for residents of their estates.

I know of a handful of health providers who include, as part of their business, a free session for beginners or those who simply cannot afford to pay. There are a lot of people in the community who do not have the luxury of being able to pay for exercise. It may be argued that keeping fit and healthy is as important for them, if not more so, as it is for those of us who can afford to pay to stay healthy.

At one of the local government programs I am currently conducting, I find the equipment freely provided by the local council is being used more than many other bits and pieces of equipment I see in my travels. I have already mentioned that free exercise equipment, as far as I have experienced, is often underused. That is, however, not the case in this instance. Perhaps it is the area where the equipment is located, or the fact that the locals are generally baby boomers. They seem to have the time to use the park. I am pleased to see what appears to be a lot of motivated locals using the provided exercise stations.

Another client of mine has recently converted his veranda into a gym. Unfortunately for me, he will no longer be coming to my sessions as often. Not only is he saving money by building his own little gym, he and his partner can choose to use it any time of the day or night. He has bought second-hand gym gear, and they now have a purpose-built facility for their own use. Initially, they had to outlay some money to buy gym equipment, albeit second-hand, but there is no further cost to be borne, at least in the short term. Perhaps you will want to do the same. The only other ingredient required, regardless of where or how much exercise costs, is motivation. Free exercise is available from many sources; you just have to be motivated to seek them out and schedule regular exercise.

I recently arranged for a client of mine to use his local park for exercise. Firstly, I had to tell him he *had* a local park. I know this may sound funny or unusual, but not everyone is completely aware of his or her surroundings. A lot of us become so busy that we miss many of the small things. I have exercised in quite a few countries around the world and, although free facilities vary from country to country, all have parks maintained at various levels that provide some exercise space.

A FEW WORDS OF CAUTION

Unfortunately, you may become sick or injured, or at the very least sore and disillusioned, at some stage during your exercise program. This is natural, and something that you will come across, even if you don't exercise. These things will happen from time to time. Not all of this will be exercise related, but no doubt some will. Do not be discouraged. Many of my clients tell me at some time or other that they feel sore, have had minor injuries or are feeling tired. This is part and parcel of exercise. In fact, it is part of life. The main thing to keep in mind is that these things are common, and although we take all measures to reduce the chances of injury, soreness and the like, they will happen. We should strive to ensure the occurrences are infrequent and minor. Keep this in mind. You need to be able to read your own body and differentiate between doing damage and simply challenging your body. Pain or discomfort is different, and you need to decide on the exercises you are doing. Decide what you can and cannot do from an exercise point of view.

Let's look at these things separately and discuss why they happen.

MUSCLE SORENESS

We in the industry, like to call this DOMS—delayed onset muscle soreness. Basically, it is soreness that has come from strenuous exercise. In most instances, it is simply an overuse of a muscle or group of muscles following an underuse situation. For example, you may start to exercise more frequently than you have in the past. You notice you have sore shoulders and biceps because you have not done body weight exercises for some time. Your muscles are not used to this. The soreness becomes apparent between 24 and 72 hours after exercise, and may be relieved with massage, stretching, warm baths and movement. Muscle soreness that does not go away after a few days should be checked by a medical practitioner, as it is possible that more severe muscle damage has occurred.

Don't be concerned about mild muscle soreness. It is quite normal. It is, however, not essential or indeed recommended that DOMS be present after every workout. Constantly having sore muscles and restricted movement is uncomfortable and does not allow us to function normally.

Although I work in the health and wellness industry, and have for some time, I still suffer DOMS from time to time, particularly after a heavy day of exercise. Be aware that you may experience DOMS when starting up an exercise program from a mainly sedentary base.

INJURIES

You may find that what you thought was DOMS was muscle damage, a tear or strain. A sprain involves overextension of a joint with stretching, and the possible tearing of a ligament. A strain is where a muscle is damaged by the tearing of tissue or tendons. Fortunately, treatment for both is similar. For minor cases, we use the acronym RICER:

- **Rest:** immobilise and rest the injured limb or area.
- **Ice:** reduces pain and restricts swelling by constricting blood vessels.
- **Compression:** apply a firm supporting bandage to the injured part.
- **Elevation:** raise the injured part above the level of the heart if possible.
- **Refer:** Get medical attention and record the details.

Of course, in the case of a more severe injury, medical attention should be sought immediately.

REST

The funny thing about rest is that often we ourselves do not recognise the signs of being tired. We rely on others to let us know. In my case, for example, my wife will tell me from time to time that I am looking tired and should rest. I am sure you have experienced similar, with someone close to you saying the same thing. Of course, we may recognise our own tiredness, but we can tend to push it to the back of our mind so we continue to finish the task at hand, or perhaps we are still at work and we have gotten used to being tired.

Being used to tiredness may be a modern malady, as we are expected to do more and more. Our balance of life, work and leisure is affected. However, the benefits of rest cannot be overstated.

I am not going to mention how many hours sleep a night you need for your body, because that will vary from person to person and also at different times in your life. Growing teenagers, for example, need more sleep to recover and feel refreshed. Your goal, in sleeping, should be to be able to perform efficiently and get through the day without major disruption from weariness.

Rest and sleep are important because these are where we recharge our batteries. The body repairs cells and tissues during sleep. Muscles may also grow. Your immune system is boosted and, believe it or not, sleep can help you lose weight. A well-rested person may act and behave more rationally, including eating sensibly. Well-rested people are often better equipped mentally and emotionally. Sleep helps us to concentrate. We all know we are in a better mood when we get enough sleep, and there are no doubt many more advantages.

From a performance point of view, it is very important that you get plenty of rest and sleep. Athletic programs for elite athletes include scheduled rest and sleep. It is so important. Once you get your program up and running and are exercising consistently, you will notice you need rest. The difference scheduling enough rest can make to your program will show you how important it is.

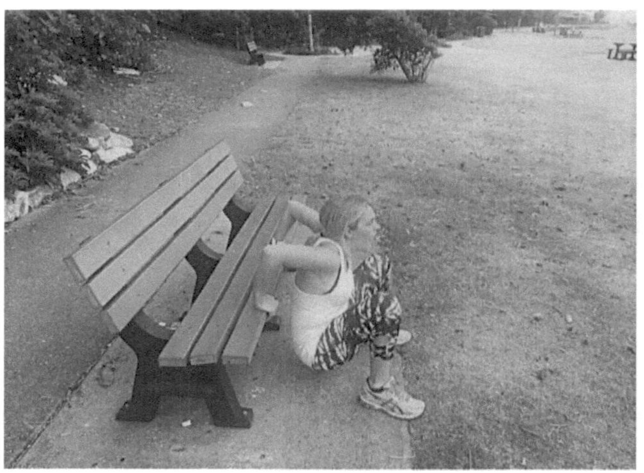

Alison improvises, using a park bench to do triceps dips.

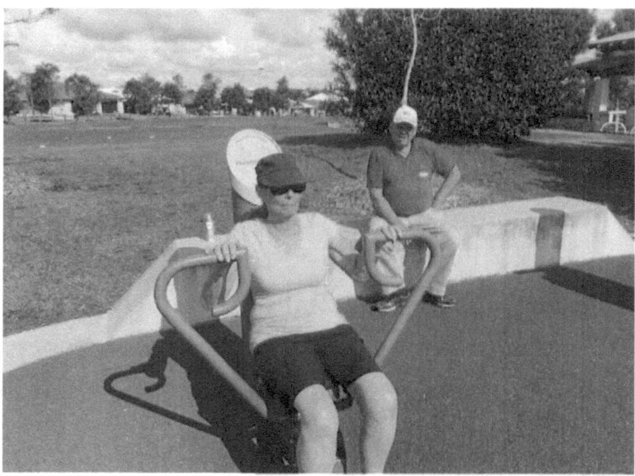

Sandra and John regularly use free park equipment in their area.

CHAPTER NINE
HOW TO NEVER DIET AGAIN

BY MITCH PETERMAN, ACCREDITED
PRACTISING DIETITIAN AND EXERCISE
PHYSIOLOGIST

Eating food is essential for human beings to stay alive. If you are lucky enough to reach 100 years of age, there is a good chance you will have consumed over 100,000 meals in your lifetime! Not only does food keep us alive, it plays an immeasurable role in our lives emotionally, socially and culturally. Indeed, eating can truly be one of life's great pleasures. Unfortunately, for many of us, deciding how to nourish our bodies can become incredibly exhausting, anxiety-provoking, time consuming and expensive.

Somewhere along the way, many of us have lost confidence in knowing how to appropriately nourish our bodies. In Western societies, this is usually driven by our fear of fat and desire for thinness. Every day, we are bombarded by messages that tell us that our worth as a human being can be defined by the shape or size of our bodies, or that there is a certain (largely unrealistic) way the human body should look.

When faced with the desire to change our bodies to become more "acceptable", many will turn to dieting. We have known for many years that dieting is a horribly ineffective way of assisting people to permanently lose weight. As this knowledge has become more common, we are seeing a rise in what I like to call "diets in disguise". These days, *diet* is considered a dirty word, so we are seeing diets being repackaged as a "healthy eating plan" or "lifestyle change". At this stage, perhaps I should be clear about what I mean when I use the word *diet*. Basically, if it tells you what to eat, how much to eat or when to eat, it's a diet. If it's a prescribed way of eating for the specific purpose of weight loss, it's a diet.

Now, it is true that some people will be successful in achieving permanent weight loss through dieting, but unfortunately these people fall into the minority. Level A evidence from the National Health and Medical Research Council (NHMRC) shows that "Weight loss following lifestyle intervention is maximal at 6–12 months. Regardless of the degree of initial weight loss, most weight is regained within a two-year period and by five years, the majority of people are at their pre-intervention body weight." So, how strong is Level A evidence? Well, it's the same level of evidence that shows that smoking causes lung cancer. Basically, we do not have an effective, safe and permanent method to help the majority of people lose weight. Now, at this stage, you may be reading with a sense of hopelessness, but do not despair. I will spend the rest of this chapter explaining how you can achieve health, happiness and contentment within your life without the need to go on a weight loss diet.

THE ART OF INTUITIVE EATING

We are all born with an innate ability to nourish our bodies appropriately. When a baby is breastfeeding, we don't have to weigh or measure the breast milk. The baby will feed until it has had enough and will let us know when it is hungry again. Miraculously, a healthy baby (free of any significant medical issues) will be nourished and grow as it should without the need for outside intervention.

Our bodies are incredibly wise. It is built into us to know when to start and stop eating, just as it is built into us to know when we need to go to the toilet when our bladder is full, to put on a jumper when we are cold or to sleep when we are tired. Unfortunately, as we grow up from being intuitively eating babies, we can begin to lose connection to our body's internal wisdom regarding how to nourish ourselves. We have so many external factors that influence our eating habits, and these can chip away at our ability to listen to our bodies and use that internal wisdom to guide our eating habits.

In simple terms, intuitive eating can be described as using internal body cues (physical hunger and fullness, feelings of satisfaction from food and how certain foods leave us feeling physically) to guide our eating behaviours. Sounds simple, doesn't it? The reality is that it can be quite a journey to effectively reconnect to these internal body cues and to redevelop the confidence to trust your body to guide your eating. After all, if you have any experience with dieting, you will realise how being on a diet encourages you to *ignore* these internal body cues and to instead eat in the prescribed way of the diet.

At this point, you may be wondering how you can start to

move away from diets and foster a healthier relationship with food through intuitive eating. For many, this process will likely involve unlearning many things that diets have taught you in the past. Patience and kindness towards yourself are important here. It may also be worthwhile engaging a dietitian who can support you to move towards becoming a more intuitive eater. To get you started on this journey, I will now outline my top ten tips for ditching the diet forever.

MITCH'S TOP 10 TIPS FOR DITCHING THE DIET

1. Strive to eat mostly based on physical hunger and fullness

When you experience cues of physical hunger (for example, a rumbly, hollow or unsettled tummy; irritability; lack of concentration; headaches or shaking), this is your body telling you that it needs some nourishment. Honour your hunger by eating! When you start to notice cues of comfortable fullness (for example, volume in the tummy; contentment; satisfaction or alleviation of physical hunger cues), this is your body telling you it has been satisfactorily nourished for now. If you are into numbers, the hunger–fullness scale below may be a useful way to think about it.

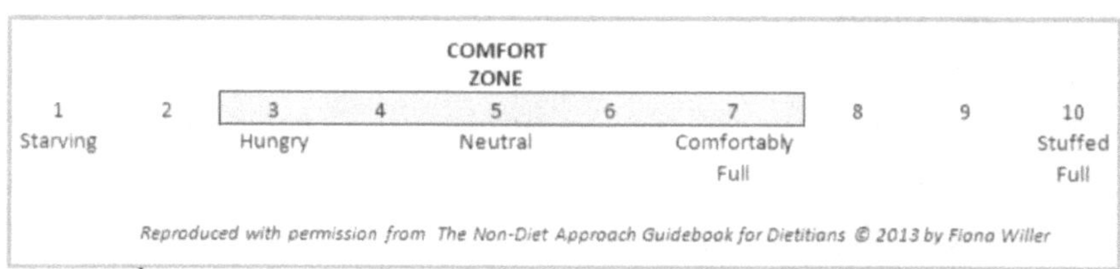

A hunger–fullness scale.

A couple of extra notes:

- Hunger and fullness can be experienced in a variety of ways. Not everyone is the same. See what you notice about your own body.
- We don't necessarily have to eat intuitively *all* the time, but we will generally feel more physically comfortable if we strive to eat intuitively *most* of the time.

2. Pay attention to how different foods leave you feeling physically

Not all foods satisfy us equally or leave us feeling the same physically. When we start to pay attention to how certain foods or meals leave us feeling physically, it can help guide our future food choices. For example, 100g of apple will leave us feeling different physically to 100g of cheese. Neither food is the right or wrong choice, but they will likely have differing effects on our perceptions of fullness and satisfaction.

3. Practise mindful eating

Practising mindfulness involves being present and attentive, in a curious and non-judgemental way. Mindfulness can be applied to anything we do, and it can certainly be applied to the act of eating. Authors have written entire books on mindful eating. It is certainly a big concept one can explore, but put simply, being mindful of when we eat can help us to better tune into our bodies and enhance the overall experience of eating. It can also help us develop a sense of gratitude for the food we are about to eat and for all the amazing steps that lead to the food or meal arriving on our plate.

To give you an idea of how to apply mindfulness in eating, when you sit down for your next meal, pretend that you are eating that meal for the first time ever. Observe its appearance with curiosity. Bring some to your nose and notice what smells you can detect. Take a bite and notice how the food feels in your mouth, what it tastes like, what the texture is like and whether there is an aftertaste. Sit with this for a moment. Was it what you expected? Did you enjoy it? Do you have a desire to eat some more? On the second or third bite, does any part of the eating experience seem different? There are no right or wrong answers here. It is simply an exercise to help you to explore your food in a more mindful way.

4. Start experimenting more with food

When we are on a diet, generally the choice of food will decrease. However, we know that the more varied our diet is, the more likely we are to meet our body's key nutrient requirements. A great way to move away from a diet mentality is to start to experiment more with foods and meals. Buy a recipe book and try cooking some new meals. Alternatively, try adding a new twist to an old favourite recipe.

5. Avoid labelling foods as good or bad, or healthy or unhealthy

Diets usually categorise foods in very black and white ways (good or bad, or healthy or unhealthy). Usually, this way of thinking doesn't help us in the long run. Food is simply food. It doesn't need to have a moral value. Let's consider chocolate cake versus a carrot. While it is obviously correct to assume they are not nutritionally equal, they are both essentially morally neutral. And if you were stranded in the desert with only water and nothing to eat other than chocolate cake, it would keep you alive.

Of course, what we eat still does matter in the long run. We don't necessarily need to be eating two serves of fruit and five serves of vegetables every day to be healthy. But to optimise our nutrition, most of us should probably be including the following foods most of the time:

- Fruits and vegetables
- Whole grains
- Milk, yoghurt and cheese (or non-dairy alternatives)
- Lean meat, chicken, fish or seafood and eggs
- Nuts, seeds and some of their oils

6. Ditch the diet talk

It's boring! Rather than talking about the latest juice cleanse diet or the supposed benefits of coffee enemas (hint: there are none), talk to people about your passions and dreams; your wonderful children; your goldfish, Fred; your recent holiday and awesome eating experiences; your favourite type of exercise or your killer business idea. When we stop giving our time and attention to diets, it frees up more time and energy for us to spend living our lives.

7. Have a social media cleanout

If you are following pages or people on Facebook or Instagram that perhaps make you feel not so great about yourself or your body, or even trigger a diet mentality, unfollow them right now. Instead, start following pages and people that promote a message consistent with a non-diet mentality. There are many out there, but a few of my favourites are:

- The Moderation Movement
- Body Positive Australia
- The Body Image Movement
- Dare to Not Diet

8. Move away from weight loss goals

As I discussed at the start of the chapter, the likelihood of permanent weight loss is not great for the majority of people. However, if we were to remove the weight loss focus, what could we focus on instead? We could consider goals that are aligned with healthy behaviours. There are quite a few key healthy behaviours that we know are important for our long-term health and well-being, and they deserve our attention. Here are some key healthy behaviours that are worth focusing on:

- eating a variety of nourishing foods, with the amount determined mainly by the body's natural hunger and fullness cues
- engaging in regular, pleasurable physical activity
- giving our bodies adequate sleep
- being socially connected
- finding enjoyable hobbies and interests
- managing stress and finding time for relaxation
- consuming little or no alcohol
- avoiding smoking and illicit drugs

9. Wear clothes you feel comfortable in right now

Embracing our bodies as they are right now can be incredibly challenging for some people. It is perfectly understandable to have a desire for our body to look different, but it can also be incredibly liberating to work towards accepting our bodies just as they are. Don't hold off on buying clothes because you are waiting until your body changes. Go out and buy clothes that look great on your body right now.

10. Strive to develop more gratitude for your body and its capabilities

The human body is truly miraculous. Think about all the things your body allows you to do, and strive to develop a sense of gratitude for your body as it is right now. Do your legs allow you to walk along the beach at sunset? Do your arms allow you to hug the ones you love? If you are a mother, did your tummy allow you to grow another human inside of you, and did your breasts provide nourishment to that little human at the start of their life?

Now think back to when you were a child. You probably didn't care what your body looked like. You probably cared that your body allowed you to run around and play with your friends. Let's fast-forward towards the later years of your life. You will again be less likely to care about what your body looks like, but more likely to care whether it helps you maintain your independence.

Developing gratitude for what our current body can do, rather than focusing on what it can't do or what it isn't, can certainly be a refreshing step in this process.

ONE LAST THING

Dieting and the relentless pursuit of weight loss can rob us of our precious time and energy, and distract us from pursuing our passions and dreams and living our lives to the fullest. So many of us put our lives on hold until we lose weight, thinking things like "I'll start dating when I lose the weight," "I'll start going to the beach again when I lose the weight," "I'll join that exercise class when I lose the weight," or "I'll start eating out with friends and family again when I lose the weight."

Newsflash! You can do all these things right now! You can do all these things in the body you currently have. Be brave and take the leap!

A final thought:

Take care of your body. It's the only place you have to live!

JIM ROHN

Mitch Peterman
www.ambitionhealth.com.au
mitch@ambitionhealth.com.au

CHAPTER TEN
THE LAST CHAPTER

If you have read this far, you are more than likely about to make some changes in how you approach your health goals and lifestyle. Well done! Nothing is perfect, but you can improve your overall well-being by adopting some of my suggestions in this book. I have no doubt your life will change for the better, in so many ways. Just imagine it now. You will have more energy. You will sleep better, you will feel lighter and happier, and you will be able to do the things you love for longer. This is not a pipe dream. It is possible. If you don't improve, because you have some injuries or illnesses that prevent you from exercising as you would wish, you will at least maintain the mobility and body functions you already have. There is a saying that the best things in life are free, and this is certainly true about keeping fit and healthy, at least in the areas we can control.

I mentioned that the last chapter would have some information to help you understand how exercise benefits you from a more technical point of view. I also want to explain some terms I have used in this book, to expand further on what they mean. You may want to delve further into this exciting time for you, and perhaps study the effects of exercise on the body further. You may be happy to simply feel better and adopt a sensible regular exercise and healthy eating program that is low maintenance and easily achieved. Regardless of how you approach your health and wellness program, some of the following information may be helpful. Don't become too concerned if you don't have the latest heart measuring device or exercise wristwatch, or you become confused about measuring a perceived rate of exertion. Tools like this are terrific and useful, but my main concern is for you to move your body more and exercise regularly. If you want to take it further by studying movement and its effects on the body, well done. The following information will help you along the way.

FIVE FREE THINGS YOU CAN DO NOW TO IMPROVE YOUR HEALTH

1. Are you still smoking? Stop now!

As mentioned previously, the science involving the body and health can and does change with further investigation and studies. One of the things that most, if not all, academics agree on is the fact that smoking is unhealthy. If you don't smoke, well done. If you do smoke, stop now. If you have tried to stop smoking in the past, and it has been unsuccessful, get some help. Hypnosis, nicotine patches, chewing gum and certainly a consultation with your doctor may assist. Whatever it takes, just stop smoking.

2. Get plenty of sleep and rest

Sleep and rest are recognised as an extremely important part of daily routine. We know that the body regenerates, heals and recharges when we sleep. Of course, from time to time we have all had periods when sleep has been irregular and insufficient, but the long-term effects of reduced sleep at the very least affect your performance in so many areas. Make sure you allocate time to get plenty of sleep and rest.

3. Mindful eating

Mitch mentions this in much more detail in chapter 9, so I will not expand more on this subject except to say that as a personal trainer, I see a lot of people who exercise regularly and appreciate, perhaps even enjoy it. Mitch invites us to be present and attentive while eating. I think chapter 9 is a great reminder to us all on how we should approach and enjoy food.

4. Alcohol

There is no way I would ever tell you to stop enjoying a drink. Drinking to excess, however, is not good for your overall health. The National Health and Medical Research Council of Australia suggests that men and women should consume no more than two alcoholic drinks on any one day. They also write, "There is no level of drinking alcohol that can be guaranteed to be completely safe or have no risk."

5. Exercise your body

I have written a great deal about this so far, and there you have it. Whatever form of exercise you choose for your regular daily or weekly regime, make sure you make it a habit if you have not already. Exercise should be second nature to you, like brushing your teeth. Keep the above five things in mind; if you can follow them, it will stand you in good stead from a health and wellness point of view.

BODY MASS INDEX (BMI)

BMI is a calculation that uses height and weight to determine your rating, be it healthy, obese or overweight. Keep in mind that ethnic and cultural differences are not taken into consideration. Variations do exist, and BMI is by no means foolproof. I consider it simply a guide, and one of many that may be used for measurement purposes. BMI is used universally as an indicator of our habits and our growing girth. The formula for calculating it is **BMI = kg/m²**, where *kg* is a person's weight in kilograms and m^2 is the square of their height in metres. A BMI of 25.0 or more is overweight, while a healthy range is 18.5 to 24.9. There is a growing trend to use waist measurement rather than BMI as a more reliable means of determining obesity.

You can find many BMI calculators on the net, where you simply punch in your weight and height and it will give you your BMI.

WAIST CIRCUMFERENCE

According to the International Diabetes Foundation, as reported by the Australian Government Department of Health, one part of the definition of "at risk" for the individual components of metabolic syndrome is **"a waist circumference**

greater than or equal to 94 cm for males, [or] greater than or equal to 80 cm for females."[1]

HEART RATE AND THE TRAINING EFFECT

When you become interested in exercise, you will be aware of terms used that reflect your heart rate: the speed at which your heart is working and how fast it is beating.

Let me explain a term we call *the training effect*. Regularly repeated physical activity produces an effect on your body that is highly beneficial to your physiological well-being; this is the training effect. All parts of your body respond positively to increased blood flow. Muscles benefit and the increase in blood assists to build and retain them. Your lungs benefit from the exercise that comes from puffing and panting. The increased flow of oxygenated blood to the vital organs not only makes you feel better, it is better for you. Endorphins produced by the central nervous system help you to feel good. They may assist in pain reduction and an overall sense of well-being. Runners often refer to a condition called *runners high*, an overall good feeling they get from consistent running, and can even experience a mild to extreme addiction to this sensation.

To take your pulse, place your index and middle finger on the carotid artery in the neck or the radial artery on the underside of your wrist for 15 seconds and multiply by four. If you assume you have a resting heart rate of 80 beats per minute (BPM), and you start a regular training program, it is more than likely your resting heart rate will lower. Resting means you have been sitting down or not doing any strenuous exercise for a few minutes.

Your heart rate can be lowered simply because you have been exercising your body aerobically. Larger volumes of oxygen being pumped around your body make your vital organs more efficient. Your heart becomes stronger, and as a result your resting pulse rate will lower. Your heart can now pump more blood around your body with less beats. Now, there is a lot more happening in the body, and all of it is generally good. In simple terms, your cardiovascular system becomes much more efficient.

MAXIMUM HEART RATE (MHR)

There are several ways of determining what your maximum heart rate (MHR) should be. Here is one of them. Keep in mind that you would first check with your doctor about exercise and physical exertion.

Start with 220 and subtract your age to calculate your MHR.

Using myself as an example: 220 – 63 years of age = 157 MHR.

This helps us to work out how intensely we have to exercise to experience the training effect. We will experience the training effect when operating at 70–80% of our MHR, which for me is around 133BPM.

Today, we have portable heart rate monitors, watches that measure our heart rate, and all sorts of devices that are extremely affordable. I still rely on measuring my clients' heart rates the old-fashioned way, by counting their pulse for 10 or 15 seconds then multiplying the count by 6 or 4 respectively. Most cardio or aerobic gym equipment has a way to measure and broadcast your heart rate, and often these machines tell you what your working heart rate should be for fitness and weight loss. Remember these readouts are a guide and may not be extremely accurate, but if you use the same machines regularly, the readout will tell you how you are doing in a relative sense.

Don't despair if you don't have a device to measure your heart rate. There is a scale called *perceived rate of exertion* or *rate of perceived exertion*. This is a numeric scale from 1–10, with 1 being very light exercise and 10 being very heavy exercise. In most cases, you should exercise at around 3–4 on this scale and increase the intensity according to your fitness levels.

Should none of the above suit, or if you simply aren't interested in recording this information, you can use the methods we have used since time began. Exercise should not injure you, but it can be uncomfortable at times. You need to learn and understand the difference between muscle soreness and damage to your body. From an aerobic point of view, you need to exercise a few times a week to the point where you feel that you are breathing more heavily and want to catch your breath. When you need to stop to catch your breath, do so, then continue on. Remember to use common sense and increase intensity and repetitions progressively.

WORK WITH A MATE

I strongly recommend you work with a mate or training buddy. The benefits of doing so are too many to mention. I will let you in on just a few. First, a mate or companion you may exercise with often feels a sense of obligation to continue to participate, as you will feel yourself. Generally, at least one of you will pick the other up and encourage them to exercise even when they may not feel like it.

Second, it is a very sensible thing to do for safety reasons. Should you have a minor accident or become injured, your mate is there to help and assist. Gentle to serious competition may result, and this can often help training partners to achieve goals more quickly than exercising alone. These are just a few reasons why finding a training partner can be so beneficial. No doubt, there are many more. Regardless, finding a training partner who is basically at the same fitness level as you is often a great move.

SAVE MONEY

You don't need the most expensive fashion brands in clothing and sporting equipment. If you have the cash and you want to, by all means get the best money can buy. In many cases, it is not necessary. Your money can be better spent on saving for a holiday or whatever else your heart desires. A pair of good walking or running shoes, some sensible light clothing suitable for the weather conditions, a cap and water bottle, and a great attitude, are really all you need. You can get reasonable quality gear by looking around and doing some research. Most stores now provide great customer service as they fight mainstream shoppers' exodus to the internet.

GOOD SHOES

I do believe you need good shoes that are appropriate for your physique and the form of exercise you have chosen. Again, this does not mean the most expensive, though good quality shoes may cost a few dollars more. I would highly recommend you get the best shoe you can. There are some speciality stores around that cater to ensuring an accurate fitting for shoes. Some use various means of discerning your gate and walking patterns. Your strike (how you hit the ground with your feet) and weight are matters a good shoe salesperson will take into consideration. You shouldn't have to spend a lot of money on good shoes, but I seriously recommend you buy good quality.

MAKE BETTER CHOICES

If you studied the life expectancy and longevity of people around the world, you would find a few things in common. First, long-lived populations are still highly dependent on movement, due to still doing some things the old way, with less reliance on new technology. Second, the way long-lived people eat and drink is generally very moderate, with a minimum of manufactured and processed foods. We also now know that stress can affect lifestyle; in some instances, depending on the type of stress, it can be very detrimental to good health. Of course, many other things may affect your overall health. Keeping healthy, eating sensibly, drinking moderately and keeping harmful stress to a minimum is a very good start.

RECORD YOUR PROGRESS OR WORKOUTS

Recording workouts using a method similar to the example log in chapter 5, helps you to keep on track. Apart from the obvious advantage that you can check on your progress, or simply that you have a record to go back to, logging is often a great motivational tool.

Recording workouts and sessions is not for everyone, and I must admit that I was resistant to recording my workouts as a younger man. However, when I started doing it, I found my logs a great tool and resource. I could look back on these records to compare my workouts over the years.

IF YOU FALTER, START AGAIN

So, you've had far too much to eat on the weekend, and drank much more alcohol than you expected. You're disappointed that your healthy eating and exercise plan has taken a hit. Don't despair. Start again! It is that simple. In fact, that is how we live our lives, if you think about it.

We get up in the morning with the best intentions of being a positive, healthy, kind, considerate person who works hard for the boss or, if you are in business for yourself, for yourself and your family. Well, I really believe and hope most of us think this way.

Richie McCaw, the famous former captain of the New Zealand national rugby union team, the All Blacks, appeared in a YouTube video before his retirement from professional football. Titled *The Game Starts Here*, it is an inspirational piece of film that presents the team, and particularly the captain, as being focused on winning and being the best they can be. In the video, McCaw gets up every morning and starts his preparation for winning.

You and I may never be as good as Ritchie McCaw, and I certainly will never be an All Black, but the message is the same for everyone. Forget disappointments, setbacks and road-blocks along your journey in life. Just start again.

Yours in health and wellness,

Tom Law OAM, Dip. Fitness
tomslaw@hotmail.com

Tom Law has been my PT and I have been a member of the Tom's Law group for almost two years. During that time, Tom has always supported me to achieve my fitness goals. Tom is ALWAYS encouraging, understanding and delivers with a good sense of humour. During the time with Tom and the group, I have lost approximately 15kg and I have gained self-confidence. Tom has trained me from being a non-runner to now preparing for half-marathon events. Over the years, I have attended many gyms and worked with numerous PTs; however, Tom Law outranks all others. He is an active community member and encourages friendships within the PT group, acknowledging all ages and fitness levels. The training environment at Suttons Beach, in the open air and amongst nature, adds to a positive training environment. Thank you, Tom!

HEATHER GIBSON

After reading this book, I started exercising more. I have never been a fan of sports, gyms, or other organised exercise activities. But I always loved walking and cycling, just to explore the world around me, and would get what I thought was plenty of exercise doing those things regularly while I lived in Australia and Japan. I have never owned a car, and always got places on foot.

Now, though, I live in a place where the outdoor environment is dangerous and unpleasant for walking and cycling. I all but stopped exercising for several years, and a lack of fitness has translated into an increased heart rate when inactive.

So I was inspired by your message that you don't need special equipment or even much space to exercise. Why had I put this off? I guess I didn't know what to do. I started off doing some jumping jacks when I would stand up to go to the toilet or make a cup of tea. Then, I discovered that I can use the emergency stairs in my apartment building to walk 16 floors up to the rooftop and back down again. I now do at least one round trip of that each day, and will build up to more as my strength improves.

Maybe I'll also come up with some other creative ideas—I am more on the lookout for exercise opportunities now since I've read *Fit Happens*.

BEN HOURIGAN

I have had the pleasure of knowing and training with Tom Law for the past few years.

As a 67-year-old working in aged care, I am well aware of the body's physical, mental and emotional needs to remain active into our later years.

Over the last few decades, I have tried to remain physically and mentally active, taking on challenges such as climbing Machu Picchu, cycling around the south of England and working in the slum areas of Africa, but I have never enjoyed the level of fitness I have gained since joining Tom's training.

I am about to walk the West Highland Way in Scotland with my 40-year-old daughter in a couple of weeks.

What I love most about Tom's training is the fun, convenience, exercising in the outdoors, the benefit of Tom's support, knowledge and expertise, and the camaraderie which comes from a team environment comprising all age groups and fitness levels.

ANNE MACINDOE, REDCLIFFE

NOTES

FOREWORD

1. A beanbag is a small material bag, about the size of a hand, filled with peas, beans or wheat, which was used to teach children how to catch, and for fun games.

WHY DID I WRITE THIS BOOK?

1. Heart Foundation, "Overweight and Obesity Statistics," https://www.heartfoundation.org.au/about-us/what-we-do/heart-disease-in-australia/overweight-and-obesity-statistics, accessed 1 August 2019.

1. SOME SCIENCE FIRST

1. Australian Government Department of Health, "Australia's Physical Activity and Sedentary Behaviour Guidelines and the Australian 24-Hour Movement Guidelines," last modified 12 April 2019, https://www1.health.gov.au/internet/main/publishing.nsf/Content/health-pubhlth-strateg-phys-act-guidelines.
2. Mayo Clinic Staff, "Exercise: 7 Benefits of Regular Physical Activity," 11 May 2019, https://www.mayoclinic.org/healthy-lifestyle/fitness/in-depth/exercise/art-20048389.
3. Kenneth Cooper, *The Aerobics Program for Total Well-Being* (Toronto: Bantam, 1982), chapter 1.
4. Australian Institute of Health and Welfare, "Life Expectancy & Deaths," last modified 28 June 2019, https://www.aihw.gov.au/reports-data/health-conditions-disability-deaths/life-expectancy-deaths/about.
5. Australian Bureau of Statistics, "4102.0 – Australian Social Trends, 2008: Public Transport for Work and Study," 23 July 2008, https://www.abs.gov.au/AUSSTATS/abs@.nsf/Lookup/4102.0Chapter10102008.

2. THE BENEFITS OF KEEPING HEALTHY

1. VO_2 max is a measurement of oxygen intake when exercising. The more oxygen consumed, the better the aerobic performance. Higher values indicate better fitness.
2. Erica M. Jackson, "Stress Relief: The Role of Exercise in Stress Management," *ACSM's Health & Fitness Journal* 17, no. 3 (May/June 2013), https://journals.lww.com/acsm-healthfitness/Pages/ArticleViewer.aspx?year=2013&issue=05000&article=00006&type=Fulltext.
3. Australian Government Department of Health, "Managing Anxiety Symptoms," June 2005, https://www1.health.gov.au/internet/publications/publishing.nsf/Content/mental-pubs-p-panic-toc~mental-pubs-p-panic-man.

3. WHAT YOU NEED TO KEEP FIT AND HEALTHY

1. Australian Government Department of Health, "Australia's Physical Activity and Sedentary Behaviour Guidelines and the Australian 24-Hour Movement Guidelines."

5. WHERE, WHEN AND HOW TO START EXERCISING

1. Mimi Spencer, *The Fast Beach Diet: The Super-Fast Plan to Lose Weight and Get in Shape in Just Six Weeks* (New York: Atria, 2014), 78.

10. THE LAST CHAPTER

1. Australian Government Department of Health, "Appendix 7. Physical Health Profile," November 11, https://www1.health.gov.au/internet/publications/publishing.nsf/Content/mental-pubs-p-psych10-toc~mental-pubs-p-psych10-21~mental-pubs-p-psych10-21-7.